MATY

Medication Administration Training for Youth

Curriculum for Participants

© VAISEF
Third Edition - 2015

Medication Administration Training for Youth (MATY) is a competency-based medication administration training program approved by the Virginia Board of Nursing. It is currently approved for use in several settings:

- Private schools and facilities licensed by the Virginia Department of Behavioral Health and Developmental Services (DBHDS), the Virginia Department of Education (VDOE), and/or the Virginia Department of Social Services (VDSS).
- Private schools that comply with the accreditation requirements set forth in Virginia statute § 22.1-19 as administered by the Virginia Council for Private Education.

The Virginia Association of Independent Specialized Education Facilities (VAISEF) has underwritten the development of this program and curriculum.

The curriculum authors are representatives from private schools for students with disabilities that are members of VAISEF.

Lisa Bales Assad LPN, BS Ed
Staff Trainer
HopeTree Family Services

Travis Baisden
Quality Assurance Coordinator
Elk Hill

Sharon Carroll RN
Health Care Coordinator
Youth For Tomorrow

Judith S. Lemke M Ed
Program Director
Inova Kellar Center

Debra Mateyka RN, BSN
Health Services Manager
Virginia Home for Girls and Boys

Kenneth Weigand Psy D
Director of Clinical Services
Timber Ridge School

First Edition published August 10, 2010.
Second Edition published November 26, 2014.
Third Edition published April 28, 2015.

The Virginia Board of Nursing approved the MATY program on January 26, 2010.
The Virginia Board of Nursing approved revisions to the MATY program on July 14, 2015.

The MATY curriculum and program are overseen by VAISEF.

Virginia Association of Independent Specialized Education Facilities
919 East Main Street
Suite 1150
Richmond, Virginia 23219
www.vaisef.org

MATY Trainers will provide education on proper and safe administration of medication, as described in the MATY Curriculum, but have no responsibility to monitor administration of medication once an individual is successfully certified through the MATY program. In the event a MATY certified medication administrator is responsible for a medication administration error, their MATY Trainer and VAISEF will bear no liability for such error. Furthermore, when an organization provides or hosts trainings for individuals other than their own employees, that organization will bear no liability for any medication errors committed by such individuals.

Table of Contents

Introduction

The purpose of this training curriculum is to provide knowledge and skills to safely and accurately administer medications to youth from infancy to age 22. This training curriculum is intended to teach staff how to assist clients in meeting their relatively common physical health care needs, such as correctly taking prescription or over-the-counter medications, communicating with licensed health care providers, and managing specific health care conditions like asthma and diabetes. Successful completion of the competency-based Medication Administration Training for Youth (MATY) means the participant learned factual information as evaluated by written tests and oral quizzes, and the participant was able to accurately demonstrate administration related procedures.

The most important teaching in MATY is **safety**. It will be emphasized and incorporated in various lessons throughout this curriculum. To ensure client safety, this training repeatedly emphasizes two essential procedures and skills: (1) always following the **Six Rights** and (2) maintaining accurate **Medication Administration Records** (MARs).

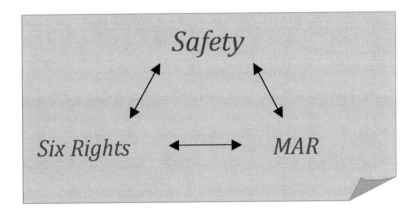

Administering medication means staff directly administer medication to clients, or staff monitor and assist clients to self-administer medications. The scope of MATY is intended to be very similar to the medication situations and needs clients have in their home and school environment.

 The hand symbol (in the left margin) is used in the MATY curriculum to emphasize the extra importance of some training information and is often related to critical safety information.

The building symbol (in the left margin) is used in the MATY curriculum to highlight information that is closely linked to the regulations, procedures, and administrative practices of individual programs. Individual facilities can and do vary in terms of specific procedures for administering medication and meeting the health care needs of children and adolescents. Therefore it is critical MATY participants know how to apply their MATY training in their particular program.

This MATY course certifies staff to administer medication to children and adolescents, as well as to assist them in self-administering medications, using the following routes.

- Oral
- Topical
- Inhaled
- Medicated Patches
- Eye
- Ear
- Vaginal
- Rectal
- Emergency injection of epinephrine using an auto-injector device
- Diabetic injections

MATY is <u>not</u>:

- intended to be a substitute for emergency medical services such as 911 community services;
- intended to be a substitute for services that should occur in an emergency room or hospital setting;
- intended to provide training to serve clients in other developmental life stages such as geriatrics or pre-school aged children;
- intended to train or empower staff to carry out procedures that require advanced education, licensing, and training such as those procedures performed by nurses, nurse practitioners, physicians, physician assistants, or pharmacists;
- intended to certify or empower staff to perform tasks beyond the scope of this training.

There are clear limits to the tasks MATY certified staff can perform under the scope of this training. Without additional appropriate training, education, and/or licensure, **MATY certified staff are <u>not</u> trained or permitted to:**

- perform medication administration duties with clients in other developmental life stages such as geriatrics in a nursing home or assisted living facility, or with pre-school aged children;
- repackage or label medications of any kind;
- administer medications that have been poured (prepared) by another person;
- pour medication for another person to administer;
- fax or call in a new prescription or orders to a pharmacy;
- write an order for, or prescribe, any kind of medication;
- give intramuscular injections (IM), including glucagon;
- teach the MATY course unless he or she meets all the trainer requirements;
- administer medication until successfully completing the entire MATY program;
- carry out procedures that require advanced education, licensing, and training such as those procedures performed by nurses, physicians, physician assistants, or pharmacists.

If a provider accepts for enrollment an individual that may need to be provided medication administration services that are not covered under the MATY curriculum, the provider should ensure that appropriate staff receive appropriate additional training to serve that individual's need.

MATY endorses a best practice approach that encompasses several trainings in order to prepare staff to meet client needs. MATY is not intended to stand alone with the skills it teaches, but should be considered an important part of a wider range of trainings and comprehensive skills that, collectively, provide safety and readiness to meet the daily needs of children and adolescents. Therefore, it is recommended that participants remain current in all of the following trainings.

1. First Aid
2. Cardiopulmonary resuscitation (CPR) and Automated External Defibrillator (AED) use
3. Standard / Universal Precautions
4. Medication Administration Training for Youth (MATY)

 When programs choose to serve clients with relatively advanced or complicated medical care needs, those programs have the responsibility to arrange for medical care that meets the clients' needs. Specifically, when facilities accept clients with significant health care needs beyond the scope of MATY, those facilities must employ staff with an appropriate level of medical training and/or provide sufficient medical care through the use of readily accessible licensed physicians, nurses or other similarly trained health care providers outside their facilities.

If training is conducted at a site other than participant's place of employment, it is recommended that they complete an orientation process at that site to translate what they have learned to their own work setting and ensure full knowledge of all program policies and procedures. Refer to Appendix 3 for a complete list of primary work place orientation items.

Section 1 – Understanding Client Rights

Participants will be able to:
- list at least three client rights related to medical care;
- list at least three of their responsibilities as staff;
- know what their obligations are when they suspect a violation of client rights has occurred related to medication administration;

Persons receiving medication and health care services have the same rights regarding their health care as anyone else not receiving services.

 Specific programs may have different ways of ethically dealing with medication refusals because medication compliance may be a requirement to receive particular services. For example, in some programs a client agrees to take medication as prescribed at the time of admission. However, no one can be forced to take medication against his or her will in the settings for which this training is intended. Be sure to review policies and procedures of your specific facility or program to determine how to address medication refusals in ways consistent with Human Rights Codes of Virginia and your program's client grievance procedure.

Client Rights Regarding Medication Administration
- Clients have the right to have their medical needs addressed in a timely fashion.
- Clients have the right to privacy. They have the right to discuss their medical concerns with staff and/or medical professionals in private. They have the right to take medications and other treatments in private.
- Clients have the right to confidentiality. Their medical information should only be shared with persons specified on a release of information form signed by a legal guardian, staff who are direct care providers, and health care providers who are connected with the program.
- Clients have the right to participate in health care decisions.
- Clients have the right to refuse medications.
- Clients have the right to be fully informed regarding medical treatment including the purpose and effects of medications, medical procedures, and tests.

Responsibilities of Staff
- Staff must respond to each client's medical needs promptly and document appropriately.
- Staff must respect a client's right to privacy during medication administration and related health care questions and discussions.
- Staff is responsible for maintaining confidentiality. Staff should discern the "need to know" before sharing information with anyone and should share medical information only with those directly involved in the care of the client.
- Staff is responsible for educating clients about their medications and side effects.
- Staff is responsible for communicating changes in behavior and/or health status to the appropriate professionals. This includes reporting medication refusals to prescribers when a pattern develops or the refusal becomes consistent.

Section 2 – Following Standard / Universal Precautions

Participants will be able to:
- explain the importance of maintaining aseptic conditions;
- identify types of body fluids;
- list necessary cleaning materials;
- state the importance of knowing where cleaning supplies are stored at their facility;
- describe how to dispose of infectious waste;
- describe proper cleaning procedures.

1. As learned in previous trainings such as Bloodborne Pathogens, Standard or Universal Precautions, and First Aid / CPR, it is important to follow precautions and procedures that reduce the chance of passing infection from one person to another. The following review of information presents steps to protect the client, staff, and others who have contact with the program.

2. Infectious waste is:

    a. any waste contaminated by an organism capable of producing disease in humans.
    b. any waste capable of producing an infectious disease in humans.

3. Always wear protective gloves when there is the possibility of touching any body fluid.

    a. Examples of body fluid
        i. blood
        ii. vaginal secretions
        iii. feces (stool)
        iv. urine
        v. vomit
        vi. sputum
        vii. nasal secretions
        viii. semen (sperm)
        ix. tears

    b. Examples of waste and materials that should be considered infectious
        i. bed linen soiled with feces, urine, or blood
        ii. containers of water used to clean infectious waste or left over residue
        iii. needles and syringes (sharps)
        iv. vials for taking blood

 4. **Staff should wash their hands** before and after all procedures. If staff's skin is touched by a body fluid, it should be washed immediately and thoroughly with soap and warm water.

5. Supplies for cleaning

   a. Bleach solution (1 part bleach to 9 parts water = 10% bleach solution)
   b. Alcohol
   c. Lysol
   d. Protective gloves
   e. Eye protection
   f. Sharps storage/disposal container (puncture resistant, leak proof)
   g. Clearly marked, leak proof, hazardous waste trash bags
   h. Paper towels

6. Staff shall be aware of where cleaning supplies are kept in the facility. Staff should visit those locations and handle the supplies to become familiar with them.

7. Important reminders about disposing of infectious waste.

   a. Disposable infectious waste should be contained in clearly marked, leak-proof plastic red biohazard bags.

   b. Needles and syringes should be placed in special red biohazard containers that are rigid, leak-proof, and puncture resistant. Sharps biohazard containers should be made of heavy red plastic. (Do not use glass or plastic beverage containers.)

   c. Contaminated water should be flushed down the toilet, and the toilet should be cleaned with a chlorine bleach solution.

8. Occupational Safety and Health Administration (OSHA) standards are periodically revised and updated. Each program should have the most current standards available and maintain compliance with those standards.

Section 3 – Medication Terminology and Abbreviations

Participants will be able to:
- identify commonly used medication and medical abbreviations;
- list the documents in which they can expect to see the abbreviations.

Knowledge of medical terminology and abbreviations is an important quality assurance tool for anyone who administers medication.

Prescriber orders and instructions written in abbreviated form will be translated by the pharmacy that fills the prescription; however, upon receipt of any new medication, the original order (when available) should be compared to the pharmacy label to check for discrepancies.

When a new medication is received, checked, and verified as accurate by the program, a Medication Administration Record (MAR) is created to list that medication information and to serve as a tracking sheet for when the medication is administered or missed. When creating a MAR, it is important to use the exact language from the pharmacy label to minimize confusion. In some instances, pharmacies will provide a ready-made MAR when a prescription is filled.

 Abbreviations should not be used on the MAR, with the exception of measurements. Measurements (such as mg and ml) are exceptions and may be used on the MAR. Staff should not use abbreviations or write in shorthand when creating a MAR. Words, numbers, times, and directions must be spelled out completely to minimize the risk of a medication error. MATY is teaching abbreviations only because they are commonly used by health care providers; therefore, staff need to be prepared to recognize and accurately decipher them.

 There are particular abbreviations that have been identified as high risk because they are too often misread or misunderstood. Difficult to understand abbreviations can result in medication errors. Appendix 6 lists abbreviations that should never be used.

Example A

The psychiatrist wrote: *Zoloft 50 mg po qd*
The pharmacy label says: Sertraline 50 mg by mouth every day

Which of the following reflects the language that should be transcribed to the MAR?
- a. Zoloft 50 mg daily
- b. Zoloft 50 mg by mouth every day
- c. Sertraline 50 mg by mouth every day

Which of these is translated incorrectly?

A more detailed learning of prescription labels and how to create a MARs will be presented later in this manual in Sections 8 and 9. See Appendix 2 for additional information and reference sources related to abbreviations and Appendix 6 for a detailed listing of abbreviations that should not be used.

 When a staff person has doubts or uncertainties about a prescription or abbreviation, the staff should always contact the pharmacy or prescriber for clarification.

Most Commonly Used Abbreviations

Abbreviation	Meaning
bid, BID	twice a day
bp, BP	blood pressure
Cc	cubic centimeter (equal to ml)
d/c, DC'd	discontinued, stopped
Gm, gm, g	gram
h, H	hour
hs, HS	bedtime (hour of sleep)
MAR	Medication Administration Record
mg	milligram
ml	milliliter (equal to cc)
NKA	no known allergies
NKDA	no known drug allergies
OTC	over-the-counter medication
oz	ounce
PCN	penicillin
per	by
po	by mouth
prn, PRN	as needed, when necessary
q, Q	every
q1h, q4h, q6h, etc.	every hour, every 4 hours, every 6 hours, etc.
qd, QD	every day, daily
qid, QID	4 times a day
qod, QOD	every other day
i, ii, iii, iiii	one, two, three, four
tbsp, T	tablespoon
tid, TID	3 times a day
tsp, t	teaspoon
WNL	within normal limits

Symbols	Meaning
△	change
↑	increase
↓	decrease
>	greater than
<	less than
#	tells pharmacist how many to dispense

Measurements	
1 cc	1 ml
1 teaspoon	5 ml = 5cc
1 tablespoon	15 ml = 15cc
1 fluid ounce	30 ml or 2 tablespoons

**Remember milliliters are liquid and milligrams are solid*

Comprehensive List of Abbreviations

Abbreviation	Meaning
ā	before
ac	before meals
APAP	acetaminophen (Tylenol)
ASA	aspirin
bid, BID	twice a day
bm, BM	bowel movement
bp, BP	blood pressure
c̄	with
Cc	cubic centimeter (equal to ml)
d/c, DC'd	discontinued, stopped
gtt	drop
GI	gastrointestinal
Gm, gm, g	gram
h, H	hour
hs, HS	bedtime (hour of sleep)
MAR	Medication Administration Record
mg	milligram
ml	milliliter (equal to cc)
NKA	no known allergies
NKDA	no known drug allergies
NSAID	non-steroidal anti-inflammatory drug
OD	right eye
OS	left eye
OU	both eyes
OTC	over-the-counter medication
oz	ounce
p̄	after
pc	after meals
PCN	penicillin
per	by
po	by mouth
prn, PRN	as needed, when necessary
q, Q	every
q1h, q4h, q6h, etc.	every hour, every 4 hours, every 6 hours, etc.
qd, QD	every day, daily
qid, QID	4 times a day
qod, QOD	every other day
s̄	without
Sig	label
sl, SL	sublingual (under the tongue)
SSRI	selective serotonin reuptake inhibitor
i, ii, iii, iiii	one, two, three, four
tbsp, T	tablespoon
tid, TID	3 times a day
tsp, t	teaspoon
URI	upper respiratory infection
UTI	urinary tract infection
WNL	within normal limits

Section 4 – Classifications of Common Medications

Participants will be able to:
- identify at least five major categories of medications;
- recall at least three generic medications and their brand names for each of the following categories - ADHD, depression, and mood stabilizers;
- define over-the-counter medications;
- define prescription medication;
- identify which categories of medications can be habit forming and/or abused by clients.
- Identify controlled substances

The classification of a medication often answers the question - What does the medication do?

Because medications may effectively treat more than one condition, some medications will have more than one classification. Occasionally a medication will be prescribed for something other than the intended use; this is referred to as "off-label use." For example, Resperidone is classified as an antipsychotic, and Valproic Acid is an anticonvulsant, but both are prescribed to children and adolescents for mood stabilization purposes.

It is important to know why a client is taking any medication. One cannot assume that the classification of a medication will always be an indicator as to why a client is taking that medication. Prescribers and other practitioners should convey the reason for administration of any medication they order for a client. If one does not know why a medication was ordered, then it is difficult to monitor the efficacy of that medication.

The following list represents several classes of medications, as well as a few specific examples of medications that may be administered to youth. This list is by no means comprehensive. It is intended to list common medications with an emphasis on psychotropic medications for children and adolescents with social, emotional, and behavioral problems. Undesired medication effects will be discussed in more detail in the next section while referring back to the table of medications.

Pill Identifier Resources: There are times in which MATY-trained staff may need to identify medications that are not in their original container or need to identify otherwise unfamiliar medications. For this reason, MATY recommends facilities are equipped with an up-to-date pill identifier book (such as the most current version of *The Pill Book*) or have on-line access to web-based pill identifier websites (i.e. Drugs.com). MATY-trained staff should never administer a medication that is not from its original packaging and most certainly never administer a medication if they are unfamiliar with its identification.

See Appendix 2 for suggested sources of comprehensive medication information.

Classification	Generic name (Trade or Brand name)	Side Effects
Attention-Deficit/ Hyperactivity Disorder (ADHD)	atomoxetine (Strattera) - non-stimulant bupropion (Wellbutrin) - non-stimulant dexmethylphenidate (Focalin)* dextroamphetamine sulfate (Adderall, Dexedrine)* lisdexamfetamine (Vyvanse)* methylphenidate (Ritalin, Concerta, Metadate)* guanfacine (Tenex, Intuniv)	Strattera: stomach upset, vomiting, dizziness, fatigue, loss of appetite, constipation Wellbutrin: worsening depression, suicidal thinking/gestures in children and teens, nausea, dry mouth, headache, blurred vision, dizziness, strange taste in the mouth, seizure ADHD stimulant medications in general: loss of appetite, weight loss, tics, abdominal pain, headache, diarrhea, mood swings, nervousness, trouble sleeping. If abused → serious heart and blood pressure problems, drug dependency or abnormal behavior
	Most ADHD medications are stimulants such as Ritalin, Concerta, Adderall, and Dexedrine; therefore, they are vulnerable to abuse by clients.	
Analgesics (pain medication)	acetaminophen (Tylenol) tramadol (Ultram) ibuprofen (Advil) hydrocodone (Lortab, Vicodin) oxycodone (OxyContin, Percocet)	Tylenol: using bruising or bleeding, new signs of infection (persistent sore throat or fever), persistent nausea, abdominal pain, rash, swelling, trouble breathing Advil: nausea, vomiting, heartburn, headache, constipation, dizziness, swelling in hands or feet, easy bruising or bleeding, difficulty swallowing hydrocodone: nausea, vomiting, dizziness, drowsiness, slow or irregular heart beat or breathing
Anti-Anxiety Medication	alprazolam (Xanax) – benzodiazepine** lorazepam (Ativan) – benzodiazepine citalopram (Celexa) – SSRI*** fluoxetine (Prozac) - SSRI paroxetine (Paxil) – SSRI clomipramine (Anafranil) imipramine (Tofranil, Janimine) busiprone (BuSpar) duloxetine (Cymbalta) venlafaxine (Effexor)	Xanax: tiredness, clumsiness, decreased appetite, nausea, confusion, slurred speech, impaired memory, rash, swelling, trouble breathing BuSpar: dizziness, drowsiness, headache, blurred vision, trouble sleeping, shakiness (tremors), muscle stiffness, jerky walking movements, rash, itching, swelling, trouble breathing, irregular heartbeat, chest pain
	**Benzodiazepine – this category of medications has a high risk for dependency and abuse.* ***SSRI – selective serotonin reuptake inhibitor. SSRIs are a relatively new class of psychotropic medications that generally increase the amount of serotonin in the brain's system, which helps treat mood disorders (such as depression and bipolar disorder), as well as anxiety. This category of medication is not habit forming and is not vulnerable to abuse. However, studies have shown that a small number of people (especially people younger than 25) who take SSRI antidepressants may experience worsening depression, other mental/mood symptoms, or suicidal thoughts/attempts. Not all antidepressant medications are officially approved for use with children and teenagers, but prescribers sometimes prescribe them because the potential benefit to an individual client is judged to outweigh the potential risk.*	
Antibiotics or Anti-infectives	azithromycin (Zithromax Z-pack) penicillin (Pen VEE-K) minocycline (Minocin)	azithromycin: upset stomach, loose stools, loss of appetite, stomach cramps, allergic reactions could include rash, swelling, trouble breathing, itching, dizziness

Classification	Generic name (Trade or Brand name)	Side Effects
Anticonvulsants	phenobarbital**** clonazepam (Klonopin) - benzodiazepine divalproex sodium (Depakote) lamotrigine (Lamictal) phenytoin sodium (Dilantin)	Phenobarbital: dizziness, drowsiness, decreased appetite, nausea, staggering or clumsiness, headache, increased dreaming/nightmares ****Phenobarbital – can be habit forming
Antidepressants	amitriptyline (Elavil) bupropion (Wellbutrin) citalopram (Celexa) - SSRI fluoxetine (Prozac) - SSRI fluvoxamine (Luvox) - SSRI paroxetine (Paxil) - SSRI sertraline (Zoloft) - SSRI	Elavil: drowsiness, dizziness, dry mouth, blurred vision, constipation, fast heartbeat, loss of appetite, weight gain, trouble urinating Prozac and Paxil: nausea, drowsiness, dizziness, anxiety, trouble sleeping, severe mood changes, uncontrolled movements or shakiness
Antipsychotics	olanzapine (Zyprexa) quetiapine (Seroquel) resperidone (Risperdal) aripiprazole (Abilify) ziprasidone (Geodon) lurasidone (Latuda) iloperidone (Fanapt)	Seroquel: constipation, drowsiness, dizziness, headache, stomach upset, nasal congestion, dry mouth, fainting, irregular heartbeat, severe mood changes, difficulty swallowing Abilify: dizziness, vomiting, blurred vision, weight gain, fast heartbeat, fainting, severe mood changes, limited facial expressions, shakiness
Antiulcer medications	famotidine (Pepcid) omeprazole (Prilosec) ranitidine (Zantac)	Zantac: headache, dizziness, constipation, diarrhea, blurred vision, easy bleeding/bruising, tiredness, irregular heartbeat
Medications for Enuresis (bedwetting)	imipramine (Norfranil, Imavate) desmopressin (DDAVP)	DDAVP nasal spray: headache, nausea, abdominal cramps, stuffy nose, nose irritation, nose bleed, sore throat
Bronchodilators	albuterol (Provental) epinephrine (Epi-Pen) montelukast (Singular)	albuterol: nervousness, shaking/tremor, mouth or throat dryness or irritation, cough, dizziness, headache, trouble sleeping, fast heartbeat, muscle cramps
Medications for Insomnia	trazodone zolpidem (Ambien) mirtazapine (Remeron) guanfacine (Intuniv, Tenex) clonidine (Catapress)	trazodone: nausea, vomiting, diarrhea, dizziness, blurred vision, weight change, dry mouth, stuffy nose, fainting, shaking/tremors, nightmares
Mood Stabilizers	topiramate (Topamax) clonazepam (Klonopin) valproic acid (Depakote) aripiprazole (Abilify) oxcarbazepine (Trileptal) lithium (Litobid) lamotrigine (Lamictal)	Topamax: fatigue, abdominal pain, poor coordination, abnormal vision, agitation, anxiety, loss of appetite, back pain, confusion, mood problems, flu-like symptoms Depakote: abdominal pain, abnormal thinking, breathing difficulty, bruising, constipation or diarrhea, abnormal mood changes, hair loss, headache, nervousness
Non-Steroidal Anti-Inflammatory Drugs (NSAID's)	aspirin (Ecotrin) ibuprofen (Motrin) naproxen (Aleve)	ibuprofen: upset stomach, vomiting, heartburn, diarrhea or constipation, drowsiness or dizziness, rash, swelling around face/tongue/throat

1. Prescription Medications

    a. Prescription medications are designated as "Controlled" and "Other."

    b. Controlled Medications (Schedule II-V)
        i. high potential for abuse
        ii. require special storage and reporting procedures
        iii. cannot be dispensed without a prescription
        iv. require consent of the client's legal guardian

    Policies and procedures related to obtaining the legal guardian's consent for medication vary from program to program.

    c. Other Medications
        i. all prescription medications not on the controlled medication list
        ii. require consent of the client's legal guardian

2. Over-the-Counter (OTC) Medications

    a. Can be administered without a prescription, but in a licensed facility, a prescriber's order is needed. In a non-licensed facility, a prescriber's order is not necessary, but legal guardian consent should be obtained.
    b. In licensed settings (private day schools or residential treatment facilities for individuals with disabilities), consent of the client's legal guardian is required to administer OTC medications.
    c. Can produce unwanted effects
    d. Examples - Tylenol, Motrin, Pepto-Bismol, B12, vitamins

3. Homeopathic and Herbal Medications

    a. MATY participants should be aware that homeopathic medications exist. They are also referred to as "remedies," "preparations," and "herbal medicines". They are often referred to as alternative or natural treatments. This category of medications is broadly defined as healing remedies that are not a part of traditional health care practices, because they have not been scientifically tested, or they have not been accepted by traditional health care practices.
    b. Programs shall seek a prescriber's advice and a prescriber's order for homeopathic medications before clients use them.
    c. A few popular examples of homeopathic medications or remedies include St. John's wort, Melatonin, Echinacea, amino acid and antioxidant supplements, ginseng, horsetail, and Calms Forte.

4. Medication Interactions – in general, it is noteworthy that the greater the number of <u>any</u> medications administered to a client, the greater the risk of adverse effects.

Section 5 – Psychotropic Medications: Purpose and Effects

Participants will be able to:
- describe the difference between desired and undesired effects of medications;
- describe the importance of observing clients for medication effects;
- describe the action to be taken when undesired medication effects are observed;
- define extrapyramidal symptoms and tardive dyskinesia;
- define a "chemical restraint" and correctly state whether it is permitted;
- identify relevant observations to be made in clinical case scenarios.

1. Desired & Undesired Effects

   a. A desired effect is favorable. It is the expected therapeutic response to the medication.

   b. Undesired effects are also called adverse effects, adverse reactions, or side effects. They are unwanted reactions to medications.

   A mild side effect is an unintended reaction to a medicine and is generally not a cause for concern. Examples of isolated mild side effects include one of the following: upset stomach; nausea; diarrhea; drowsiness; irritability; headache; trouble sleeping.

    An adverse effect is unexpected and more serious. Notify the prescriber and the legal guardian. Call 911 if the adverse effect or reaction is severe or potentially life threatening. Examples of adverse effects are repeated vomiting, severe dizziness, chest pain, seizures, and difficulty breathing. Adverse effects can also include highly unusual changes in mental status or behavior, such as disorientation, confusion, odd speech patterns, seeming out of touch with reality, or high levels of energy and agitation.

   Review undesired effects in the table of medication information listed in Section 4.

   c. Extrapyramidal Symptoms

   Extrapyramidal symptoms are neurological side effects of antipsychotic medication. Symptoms can occur within the first few days or weeks of treatment, or it can appear after months and years of antipsychotic medication use.

   Extrapyramidal symptoms are more common among clients taking conventional antipsychotic medications compared to the newer atypical medications that are often used as mood stabilizers in children and adolescents. Extrapyramidal symptoms can cause a variety of symptoms such as involuntary movements, tremors, rigidity, body restlessness, muscle twitching or contractions, and changes in breathing and heart rate.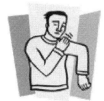

d. Involuntary Movements (Tardive Dyskinesia)

One of the most common extrapyramidal symptoms is involuntary movements most often affecting the mouth, lips, and tongue. For example, clients may have facial tics, roll or repeatedly protrude their tongue, or lick their lips. Sometimes the trunk or other parts of the body are also affected. This side effect is usually managed or minimized by reducing the medication dosage or by changing type of medication; however, the symptoms may persist even though the medication is altered.

Observe clients closely anytime a new medication is begun. **If any of the symptoms listed above develop, contact the prescriber immediately.**

e. All medications have side effects. Therefore, it is important to know how to access additional detailed information when needed. The information sources and references listed in Appendix 2 are commonly seen as legitimate, accurate, and helpful, but MATY does not intend to endorse any particular book or internet site. Please also pay attention to pharmacy inserts.

2. Reporting physical, emotional, cognitive, and behavioral changes is an important responsibility of direct care staff. Staff's role is to constantly observe. Undesired effects should be reported to the correct person, at the correct time, in the correct way, using the correct channel according to the procedures and regulations of the program.

3. Documentation will be discussed in more detail in Section 9, but it is noteworthy at this point to introduce and highlight the importance of thorough documentation by staff. Documentation is critical because:

a. a permanent record is required by federal and/or state regulations;

b. client observations may be required by the program;

c. observations are critical to tracking progress during treatment and schooling, otherwise client goals and objectives cannot be evaluated;

d. it helps the prescriber evaluate whether medication is effective or not;

e. it keeps staff focused on the needs, strengths and problems of an individual client;

f. when problems arise, the "paper trail" of documented observations can be extremely helpful in pinpointing what might have gone wrong for a client;

g. when successes occur, the paper trail of observations can be used to help pinpoint what interventions tend to work best for an individual client;

h. it is one means by which staff persons communicate with each other about a client to provide a continuum of care, to help the client progress no matter which staff are working on a particular day or shift;

i. it is a means by which precautions can be put in place for a client, if he or she needs to avoid certain medications or foods due to adverse reactions in the past.

4. Chemical Restraints

   a. Chemical restraint is a term used to describe giving a client medication with strong sedating effects to calm him or her down when extremely agitated.

   b. For the purpose of working with clients described in this MATY curriculum, <u>chemical restraints are never permitted</u>.

5. Clinical Case Examples for Psychotropic Medications

   Read and discuss each of the following case scenarios. Consider what kinds of observations should be made when documenting notes of each of the teenagers. Consider the desired therapeutic effects that might occur and consider the mild unwanted side effects, or adverse effects, that should be monitored.

   a. Manuel is a 13-year-old in the 6th grade. He was recently admitted to a residential facility a few weeks after the Department of Social Services (DSS) had to assume custody of him because his parents were experiencing severe substance abuse problems and legal troubles. Emotionally, Manuel was experiencing a mix of anger toward his parents, fear he might never be reunited with them, and sadness over the situation. He displayed extremely uncooperative behaviors when initial attempts were made to place him with a foster family, and the few extended family members in the area were unwilling to take care of him. The residential facility staff observed that Manuel was very critical of himself, irritable, and talked in hopeless ways about his future. They also observed and documented that his appetite was declining. In addition, Manuel's therapist administered psychological testing that revealed high scores on measures of depression and oppositional behaviors. Records from a previous school counselor revealed Manuel's academic performance had been suffering the previous couple of years, and staff was worried that he worked too hard to cover up depression and worries about his home situation by acting overly tough and macho. Based on this information and an interview with Manuel, his psychiatrist started him on a prescription for Prozac, an SSRI antidepressant.

      • What problem behaviors should staff persons be alert for when working with Manuel?
      • What medication side effects should staff persons monitor?
      • What possible improvements should staff be monitoring and documenting?

b. Stephen is a 15-year-old who is a 9th grade student in a day school program that offers special education services. Staff report in a treatment team meeting that Stephen is "hyper" and gets into the business of other students frequently. The teacher observes that Stephen can barely stay focused on assignments for 5 minutes, and his school papers and notebooks are messy soon after he gets them organized. Other staff notice that for his age, he has trouble waiting his turn like a much younger student might and interrupts others routinely. ADHD is not a surprising diagnosis for Stephen. The psychiatrist recently increased Stephen's dose of Adderall from 5 mg at 8:00 am and 12:00 noon to 10 mg at 8:00 am and 12:00 noon.

- What possible improvements should staff be monitoring and documenting?
- What medication side effects should staff monitor? (see Section 4)
- What problem behaviors should decrease for Stephen in the near future due to the increase in Adderall dosage?

c. Rebecca is a 15-year-old honor student in the 9th grade at a short-term residential facility. Despite her above average intelligence and the fact she is generally well liked by her peers, she sets excessively high expectations for herself. She worries frequently about "getting things right" to the point she obsesses and has unwanted intrusive thoughts about being perfect. Her intense worrying over details interferes with completion of her school work, having spontaneous fun with others, and being on time with her morning routine before breakfast. In the past, "perfect" for her often meant extremely clean, so she engaged in long periods of hand washing, which decreased her worrying for a short while. Her diagnosis is Obsessive-Compulsive Disorder. The psychiatrist recently started Rebecca on Paxil to treat the anxiety based problems and in part chose that particular SSRI medication because Rebecca's mother had a good response to it for similar, but less severe, problems a few years ago.

- What behavioral and thinking improvements should staff persons be looking for in Rebecca given her medication?
- What problem behaviors should staff monitor?
- What possible side effects should staff be watchful for in case Rebecca experiences adverse effects? (see Section 4)

Section 6 – The Six Rights of Medication Administration

The participants will be able to:
- list the Six Rights of medication administration;
- understand how to use the Six Rights to administer medication correctly;
- identify the conditions necessary for safe medication administration.

A. The Six Rights of Medication Administration

1. **Right Client**
2. **Right Medication**
3. **Right Time**
4. **Right Dose**
5. **Right Route**
6. **Right Documentation**

Each time you administer medication make sure to follow the Six Rights.

B. Right Client

Staff must **always** be certain the medication is administered to the correct client. This can be done by confirming one or more of the following.
- asking for his or her name
- checking a wrist band
- having another staff present to confirm the client's name
- asking for individualized information such as date of birth or allergies
- looking at client pictures kept in the medication administration area

Do not allow yourself to feel too embarrassed when asking a client his or her name, or for his or her identifying information. It is the best practice to follow no matter how you feel and could prevent a serious error.

C. Right Medication

To make sure you give the right medication use the following process.

a. Compare the prescriber's order and Medication Administration Record (MAR) to the pharmacy label.

b. Make sure the MAR and pharmacy label agree. If they do not agree, contact your supervisor for further instruction. Do <u>not</u> administer medication when the MAR and pharmacy label do not match.

D. Right Time

When a prescriber orders a medication, he or she will specify how often and when the medication should be taken.

As a reminder, MATY does not endorse abbreviations. Staff will see abbreviations written by health care providers; therefore, the following is intended to be a brief refresher from abbreviations listed in Section 3.

QD	Once a day		Q 8 hrs	Every 8 hours
BID	Twice a day		QAM	Every morning
TID	Three times a day		QHS	Hour of sleep
QID	Four times a day		ac	Before meals
Q6h	Every 6 hours		pc	After meals

 There is typically a "window of time" in which a prescribed medication can be given safely and appropriately. Instructions from the pharmacy or attending prescriber supply this information. As a general guideline, the window of time medications can be administered is one hour before, and one hour after, the time designated on the prescription and the pharmacy label.

 It may be common practice for staff to travel with a client off-site. Staff should therefore check in advance and verify if a student has a prescribed medication that will need to be administered during the time away from the facility. Procedures will vary from facility to facility; however, staff are expected to know their individual facility's procedures for on-time administration of medications when off-site with a client. Those off-site procedures will generally include the following steps.

1. Plan ahead to allow sufficient preparation time before going off-site to arrange a vehicle, gather travel directions, gather necessary paper work, communicate with other staff about the pending departure, and to gather medications during the time away period.

2. In situations where two or more staff will be traveling with a group of clients, staff should communicate clearly among themselves who will be the lead certified medication administration person to gather, store, hold and administer medications during the off-site trip.

3. Without delay, medication administrations should be recorded using proper documentation procedures after returning to the facility.

E. Right Dose

Compare the prescriber's order and MAR with the pharmacy label to make sure they agree. Carefully measure or count the correct dosage. Do <u>not</u> administer medication when the prescriber's order and MAR dosage and pharmacy label dosage do not match.

<u>Titrating</u>

Pay careful attention to directions involving titration, when a medication dosage is gradually increased or decreased to alleviate possible side effects and/or to reach a therapeutic level of a medication.

> Example of titrating down
> > Prednisone 20 mg – 2 tabs by mouth, 2 times a day for 3 days, then decrease
> > Prednisone 20 mg – 1 tab by mouth, 2 times a day for 3 days, then decrease
> > Prednisone 20 mg – 1 tab by mouth, once daily for 3 days, then stop.

> Example of titrating up
> > Depakote 250 mg – 1 tab by mouth, 2 times a day, for 10 days, then increase
> > Depakote 500 mg – 1 tab by mouth, 2 times a day, for 10 days, then increase

F. Right Route

There are nine routes used for medication administration.

1. Oral
2. Topical
3. Nasal
4. Eye
5. Ear
6. Parenteral
7. Injection
8. Rectal (per facility regulations and policy)
9. Vaginal (per facility regulations and policy)

Never crush a pill without a doctor's order. Be aware that a pill crushing device should not be used to crush more than one type of medication.

Never split a pill in half, which is not scored. A scored pill is manufactured with a line across the mid-section to make it easier to break into two equal halves. Pill splitting devices exist and are recommended in order to carry out this task precisely.

Staff should always compare and verify the route in the prescriber's order matches the route listed in the MAR and on the pharmacy label. Do <u>not</u> administer medication when the route indicated in the prescriber's order and MAR route and pharmacy label route do not match.

G. Right Documentation

Each time a medication is administered to a client, the medication, date, time, dose, route, person administering medication, and client name must be accurately recorded in the MAR without delay. In addition, document any side effects. Section 8 and Section 9 present detailed information on documentation, as well as opportunities to practice creating a MAR and writing MAR entries.

H. Other Important Considerations

Avoid distractions when giving out medications. A high level of activity or noise can cause staff to make a mistake, even when a staff person knows the client well.

Even though medications can be given for long periods of time, there is always a possibility that a change has been made. Double check all Six Rights every time you administer a medication.

Section 7 – Accessing, Maintaining and Sharing Medical Records

Participants will be able to:
- demonstrate how to access and read client medical records;
- demonstrate how to access and read vital information such as information about current medication or other allergies, current medications, and the names and contact information of a client's physician, dentist and medication prescriber;
- find and list key points in the facility's regulations and policies regarding medical and dental records;
- list the information necessary to provide to a physician, dentist or prescriber when accompanying a client to a medical or dental appointment;
- list the information that should be received from a physician, dentist or prescriber at the conclusion of a medical or dental appointment.

When participants receive MATY training at a site that is not their primary work place (i.e., away training at a host facility), they may have access to client medical and/or dental records and medication administration areas at the training site through trainer lessons or demonstrations. In these situations, and any other situation in which confidential information is exposed, MATY participants are expected to uphold client confidentiality standards by keeping private information private.

1. Discuss procedures for storing medical and dental records. Topics and activities include:

   a. discussing whether records are kept electronically, in paper files, or a combination of both;

   b. describing what information is required for admission or enrollment in the program;

   c. describing how and where to access the medical and dental records;

   d. having the trainer demonstrate how to actually access the electronic or paper records;

    e. having the trainer point out where specific pieces of information can be found such as:

        i. current medication or other allergies
        ii. current medications
        iii. medical history and dental history
        iv. most recent physical and dental exam
        v. copies of physician, dentist's and prescriber orders
        vi. copies of prescriptions
        vii. contact information for current physician, dentist and prescriber
        viii. contact information for client's legal guardian if he/she is a minor
        ix. contact information for the client's placing or referring agency if applicable
        x. descriptive information of client's recent adjustment related to mental and physical status
        xi. "permission to treat" form signed by the legal guardian (when applicable for minors in your care)
        xii. up-to-date insurance coverage information

2. Participants should be able to describe how and where to access the facility's policies, regulations, and memos related to maintaining and sharing the client's medical and dental records.

3. Read and discuss the facility's written regulations, policies, and memos for accessing, maintaining, and sharing medical and dental records.

4. When a staff person accompanies a client to an appointment with a physician, dentist or prescriber, the following information should be <u>taken to the appointment</u>.

    a. a copy of relevant medical records for the first appointment or current vital information (not the original medical record)
    b. history of medication or other allergies
    c. current medications and reasons they are given
    d. current medical and dental conditions not being treated with medication
    e. name and contact information of treating physicians, dentists or prescribers
    f. written observations of the client's mental, behavioral, and physical status noting recent changes, if any

5. When a staff person accompanies a client to an appointment with a physician, dentist or prescriber, the following information should be <u>received from that provider</u> at the conclusion of the appointment.

    a. medication ordered (name, form, strength, daily dosage and count)
    b. purpose and desired effect of medication
    c. unwanted effects or side effects that should be monitored (as discussed in Section 5)
    d. possible interactions with other medications the client is currently taking
    e. medications that should be discontinued when the new one is started
    f. special storage and/or administration instructions

6. Case Scenarios for Group Discussion

   a. At his residential facility, Timmy (age 12) has recently begun to wet the bed at night. The night staff notified the treatment team including the facility's nurse. One part of the treatment team's response is to schedule a medical consultation with a pediatrician, so that possible physical reasons for the nocturnal enuresis can be evaluated. The staff person who accompanied Timmy to his first appointment with the pediatrician brought along a copy of Timmy's complete medical history prior to entering the residential facility. What other information should have been brought for the pediatrician?

   b. Michelle (age 13) attends a day school. Her mother (legal guardian) informs the day school staff that Michelle was prescribed Zoloft by her psychiatrist the previous day. The mother then hands the staff (1) a copy of the prescription, (2) a copy of the psychiatrist's order, and (3) a properly labeled bottle of Zoloft she had just picked up from the pharmacy. What else does the staff person need to know? What else does he or she need to consider? What action should he or she take?

   c. David (age 15) has been in your residential facility for 6-months. As a full-time staff person, you know David well. Your supervisor asks you to transport David for an updated and required physical exam at the physician's office. As you prepare for the trip, you are told your facility's nurse is unexpectedly absent from work today due to a family situation of some kind, and the paperwork that would normally be gathered by the nurse and handed to you is not available. You must leave for this hard-to-get appointment in 30 minutes. What do you do?

   d. You are a staff person at a day school. One of the clients in your care is Marrissa (age 10) who resides in a group home when she is not at your day school. The Department of Social Services is the legal guardian. When Marrissa fell on the playground during recess time today, you accompanied her to the urgent care clinic when it was suspected she may have fractured her arm. You brought all the correct paperwork, and the examination was completed by the physician. They brought Marrissa back out to you in the waiting room and said, "She is fine. She is ready to go. Maybe give her some ibuprofen in a couple hours." However, it does not look as if the urgent care staff are going to hand you any paperwork or documentation at all on your way out. What should you do?

Section 8 – Medication Administration Records (MARs) and Other Medication Forms

Participants will be able to:
- accurately decipher a prescription;
- accurately decipher a prescriber's order;
- accurately read and interpret a pharmacy label;
- accurately read and interpret an over-the-counter (OTC) label;
- thoroughly understand a MAR.

1. It is important that staff accurately understand and complete the various forms related to medications, so that clients receive medications and treatments as the prescriber intends. Staff should be thoroughly familiar with the process from start to finish, from the time a prescription is written, to the time of recording that the client received the medication, to the time of recording whether there were desired or undesired medication effects.

2. Staff should be comfortable and familiar with how to read prescriptions, the information contained in a prescriber's order, how that information is conveyed in a pharmacy label, and how that information is transferred on to a MAR. The MATY certified staff has the responsibility of knowing how to verify that all of this information is consistent to ensure the well-being of the client.

3. The following are standard elements of a prescription.

   a. Prescriber contact information

   b. Drug Enforcement Agency (DEA) number

   c. Name and contact information of patient

   d. Date

   e. Medication dosage

   f. Medication route

   g. Medication frequency

   h. Date of discontinuation or length of time the medication is to be given if applicable

   i. Number of refills

   j. Number of pills/capsules

Written Prescription Example

> **John Adams, M.D.**
> 123 Elm Street
> Anywhere, Virginia 23200
> (804) 333-5555
>
> DEA # 12345678
> ===
>
> **Name:** John Doe   **DOB:** 1/1/2000
> **Address:** 456 Main Street
>   Richmond, Virginia 23200
>
> **Rx**
> *Adderall 10 mg #30*
>
> *1 tab po qam*
>
>   Refills: 0 1 ② 3 4 5
> ☐ Dispense as written
> ☐ Voluntary formulary permitted
>
> _____ M.D.
>
> *if neither box is marked, a voluntary*
> *formulary product must be dispensed.*

4. <u>Prescriber's order</u>. There is no single format or form used by prescribers to write medical treatment orders. But, prescriber orders usually contain the same bits of information, such as:

    a. Client's name
    b. Client's date of birth (DOB)
    c. Allergies
    d. Current date
    e. Treatments that may not include medication
    f. Medications – listing necessary prescription information
    g. Prescriber's signature
    h. Possibly the client's facility name
    i. Possibly the client's insurance/Medicaid number

5. <u>Pharmacy labels</u>. The following are elements of the pharmacy label.

    a. Client's first and last name
    b. Authorized prescriber's name
    c. Pharmacy name and contact information
    d. Date prescription was filled
    e. Name of the medication
    f. Dosage of the medication
    g. Route of the medication
    h. How often to give the medication
    i. Date the medication is to be discontinued or length of time in days the medication is to be given, if applicable
    j. Number of pills/capsules
    k. Number of refills

Pharmacy Label Example

```
                        ABC Pharmacy
                        1234 Main Street
                    Crossroads, Virginia 23100
                        (540) 333-5555
    ==================================================
    Rx 789-654                              Date 5-20-15


    Thomas Hyperson


    Tabs. Adderall 10 mg #30
    Take one (1) tablet by mouth every morning



    Refills:  0  1  ②  3  4  5          John Adams, M.D.
```

6. <u>Over-the-Counter (OTC) Medication Labels</u>. OTC medication must be in its original container and be labeled with the client's first and last name, unless it is house stock that anyone can use after physician (or guardian) approval.

Common and important information on OTC labels include:

   a. Active ingredients
   b. Uses
   c. Warnings
   d. Directions
   e. Other information
   f. Inactive ingredients
   g. Contact information for questions or comments
   h. Expiration date

7. <u>Medication Administration Record</u> (MAR)

 Each facility may be different in the forms it uses for the required documentation related to medication and medical records. MAR forms are no exception, but below is a list of what should appear on all MARs in some format or another.

   a. Name of the client
   b. Name of the medication
   c. Dosage of the medication   **Five of the Six Rights**
   d. Time(s) to be given
   e. Route of administration
   f. Special instructions for storage or administering (if applicable)
   g. Place for each staff to provide legible signature and corresponding initials
   h. Place for initials of identified staff each time medication is administered
   i. Place for noting when medication was not given
   j. Place for noting error
   k. Place for noting why a prn medication was given and its effectiveness
   l. Start date
   m. Stop or discontinuation date
   n. Special instructions for storage or administering (if applicable)

Additional samples of MARs are located in Appendix 9.

Section 9 – Documenting Medication Administration

Participants will be able to:
- identify reasons for keeping a record of medication administration;
- identify what information should be documented on a MAR;
- demonstrate accurately creating a MAR;
- demonstrate accurately making MAR entries;
- demonstrate accurately making an "as needed" (prn) medication entry;
- accurately state the difference between describing a client versus diagnosing a client when communicating verbally or through written documentation.

1. Best practice and required procedures include:

    a. Documenting all medication administered (even OTC medication);
    b. Using the appropriate MAR per each client;
    c. Documenting immediately after giving medication;
    d. Documenting in ink;
    e. Writing legibly;
    f. Documenting side effects;
    g. Documenting exactly what was seen to necessitate an "as needed" (prn) medication.

2. **Each time** a medication is given to a client, the medication name, dose, date/time, route and name of the client must be recorded. Also, the staff person's initials must be recorded on the MAR each time a prescription or OTC medication is administered. The full signature is usually located elsewhere on the MAR.

3. Documenting medication administration helps to prevent medication errors and helps maintain a routine pattern of administering medications on a daily basis so the medications are received as prescribed.

4. If an error is made making a MAR entry, cross out the incorrect information with a single line and write "error" and your initials next to it. Never use white out.

MARs are legal documents and need to be kept on file for at least three years after the client leaves the program. Individual facilities and programs are responsible for knowing and complying with state regulations pertaining to maintenance and storage of client records.

When making MAR or medication related entries in other records of the client (such as progress notes), staff should document observations and descriptions of clients, but never make diagnoses or use diagnostic phrases unless licensed and credential to do so.

- For example, it is appropriate to document that a client's facial expression appears sad, that the client appears lethargic, or that a client has been tearful. But it is not acceptable for staff to document that a client is suffering from depression, because depression is a diagnostic category, and it is a conclusion about the client.

- For example, it is appropriate to document that a client seems unable to sit still for longer than 5 minutes, that he interrupts other people's conversation approximately 4 times every hour, and that he very often touches things impulsively. But it is not acceptable for staff to document that a client has Attention-Deficit/Hyperactivity Disorder (ADHD) because ADHD is a diagnosis.

- For example, it is appropriate for staff to document that a client sounds congested, has a temperature of 101 degrees, and she states that she did not eat at lunch or dinner because she did not feel hungry. It is not appropriate for staff to communicate that the female client has the flu or possible viral infection because those are diagnostic categories and conclusions about a client's health.

See Appendix 4 for a list of client descriptions that could be used to help communicate useful clinical information.

Home Visit

Home visit reflects when a client is sent on a home visit, for a day pass, overnight visit, or extended home pass. All medications will be sent home in the original packages.

To document on the MAR, write HV with a circle around it each time the client is going to take that particular medication at home, and document, usually on the back of the MAR, the names of the medications packed and sent home.

Section 10 – Documenting Medication Errors

Participants will be able to:
- describe why documenting medication errors is important;
- list the information that should be contained in a medication error report;
- list common reasons for medication errors;
- demonstrate they can complete a medication error report competently.

1. The goal is to have zero medication errors to ensure client safety, as well as effective treatment. In the interest of safety and the prevention of future problems, it is important to know about medication errors and their details as soon as they are recognized.

2. Medication error reports <u>must be completed</u> when medication errors occur.

3. A medication error is usually defined by situations in which one or more of the "Six Rights" went wrong. (Reminder, the Six Rights are Right Client, Right Medication, Right Time, Right Dose, Right Route and Right Documentation.) Other examples of medication errors include when staff forget to administer the medication, the medication is expired, or it is given without a prescriber's order.

4. Again, forms vary including medication error reports, but the content and information required in those reports include, but are not limited to, the following.
   a. provider or facility name
   b. facility address and phone number
   c. client's name
   d. client's date of birth
   e. date and time of medication error
   f. type and details of medication error; why and how did it occur?
   g. action taken (examples include notification of guardian/parent, notification of prescriber, increased monitoring of client, providing or arranging for medical care due to the error, calling poison control)
   h. corrective action to be taken in the future (re-education of staff, for example)
   i. name of person completing medication error report
   j. date medication error report completed

5. Facilities should have policies and procedures for when a medication error occurs:
   a. Notification of prescriber
   b. Notification of parent/guardian
   c. Internal supervisory review
   d. Corrective action procedures

6. If the medication error involved more than one client, then one medication error report should be completed for each client.

7. One avoidable medication error is running out of the OTC or prescribed medication. Medication quantities should be routinely monitored. When medications begin to run low, they should be replenished in a sensible amount of time that prevents running out of the medication completely.

Section 11 – When Clients Refuse Medication

Participants will be able to:
- understand and anticipate that clients sometimes refuse medications;
- list reasons why clients might refuse medications;
- identify the most important staff responses when a medication is refused;
- describe at least three staff interventions aimed at resolving the situation;
- correctly state whether or not a client can receive a negative consequence (i.e., behavioral punishment) for refusing his or her medication;
- identify deceptive behaviors sometimes shown by clients.

Children, adolescents, and young adults sometimes refuse to take prescribed medications. This situation should be expected by staff from time to time, and it may occur with some regularity with particular clients given their social, emotional, and behavioral problems. Although specific procedures may vary among programs, there is a sequence of steps that should generally be taken.

1. **Listen to the client.** This is the most important response staff should take. Do not assume that he or she is simply being defiant or uncooperative for no good reason. Listen to what the client is saying about his or her medications in order to find out what is motivating him or her to refuse medications. There are several important possibilities to listen for, such as:

   a. the client may be experiencing unwanted or unpleasant side effects (i.e., adverse effects) that require medical attention;

   b. the client might have distorted beliefs or misunderstandings about the purpose of the medication, the need for it, or its potential adverse effects;

   c. the client may have realistic or unrealistic fears;

   d. the client may have had adverse reactions to other medications in the past and is emotionally recalling that similar experience;

   e. the client might not want to miss out on activities with other children or teenagers so he or she is refusing to take the time to take the medication;

   f. the client may still be upset about a social situation that occurred a short while earlier, and he or she is now acting out for no reason directly related to the medication;

   g. It may be a new medication for the client, and he or she needs extra time, support, and information before agreeing to take it as prescribed.

2. **Take action.** No matter what the client's reasoning and behaviors for refusing the medication, take action. The most appropriate action obviously depends upon the client's reasoning.

   a. Based upon training and active listening skills, if staff believes the client is experiencing adverse reactions to a medication, immediately notify the attending health care professional such as the prescriber or the program's or facility's nurse and convey the information. The Poison Control hotline is another alternative depending upon the situation. Clients are often minors, so staff should also contact the legal guardian about the situation. Depending upon the client's family situation, there may be a parent figure that should be notified, even though the parent figure may not be the legal guardian.

   b. Based upon training and active listening skills, if staff determines the client's refusal is <u>not</u> related to adverse reactions or medical problems, staff should utilize their interpersonal childcare skills to resolve the emotional or behavioral causes of the refusal. Options for specific interpersonal interventions include:

      i. Allowing the client time and space to calm down, which often leads to better judgment and thinking.

      ii. Calmly communicate to the client about why the medication is being prescribed, why it is important to take it as prescribed, and the possible medical or emotional or behavioral problems that may worsen if the medication is not taken.

      iii. Spending time with the client to educate him or her about the "right way" to discontinue medications, which is to talk with the prescriber at the next medication appointment about the reasons for wanting to stop the medication. In a supportive tone, reminding the client that some medications require time to slowly and safely discontinue them, and that suddenly stopping the medication could cause worse medical or emotional problems.

      iv. Helping the client to resolve the emotionally upsetting problem that is occupying their attention so he or she can then move forward with taking the medication within the prescribed period of time.

3. **Notify.** If the above interpersonal interventions do not work after a period of time, staff should follow the facility's procedures related to notifying appropriate persons about missed or refused medications. Depending upon the individual facility's regulations and possible prescriber guidelines, the list of appropriate persons to notify could include the facility's supervisory staff, the prescriber, legal guardian, parents, and agency persons involved with the client (such as the client's social worker).

4. **Document.** When clients take their prescribed medication, it must be documented. When clients refuse to take their medication or if there if a medication error, it must be documented.

5. **Do not punish.** Client rights and quality care practices require that clients not receive negative consequences for refusing medication. Refer back to Section 1 to review information regarding client rights.

6. **Deceptive client behaviors.** There is always a degree of risk for children and adolescents (especially those who exhibit social, emotional and behavioral problems) to be manipulative, sneaky or deceptive with their medications. For example, deceptive clients may attempt to "cheek" their medications by not actually swallowing pills or capsules they put into their mouths. For various reasons, deceptive clients may attempt to subtly grab and hide medications within their reach during medication administration time. Therefore, it is extremely important for staff to be vigilant in storing, monitoring and administering medications.

   One specific practice that should be followed routinely is a "mouth check" when administering oral medications (i.e., pills, capsules, caplets). A mouth check is when clients are asked to open their mouths and lift their tongues immediately after swallowing a pill, while staff visually inspect for hidden pills along their gum lines or under their tongues. Another specific and routine practice during medication administration is for staff to not keep medications within reach of clients, and to not turn their backs on clients in the medication administration area.

Section 12 - Pouring and Preparing Liquid Medications

Participants will be able to:
- explain and/or demonstrate the correct procedure for administering oral liquid medication.

1. When preparing liquid medication, follow the steps below.

    a. Wash hands.

    b. Identify the desired measurement from the doctor's order or the MAR.

    c. Shake medicine, per label instructions, if applicable.

    d. Pour the medication to the desired level making sure the medicine cup is on a flat surface.

    e. Always bring your eye to the same level as the medicine cup.

    f. If too much was poured, or if the client refuses the medication after it is poured, discard the excess. Do not pour the medication back into the bottle.

2. When administering the liquid medication, follow the steps below.

    a. Hand medicine cup to the client and watch him or her drink the medicine.

    b. Add a small amount of water to the medicine cup and ask the client to finish what may have been left over.

    c. Offer water to the client.

3. Do not substitute household items, such as household baking spoons, kitchen teaspoons, or measuring cups for dosing devices. Graduated health care measuring instruments that are intended for liquid measures should be used.

4. Due to the potential for error, you should never convert a dose from one measurement to another.

Section 13 - Measuring and Recording Vital Signs

Participants will be able to:
- identify normal ranges of vital signs;
- competently measure a person's vital signs;
- record vital signs appropriately.

Normal measurements for each client vary. It is always a good idea to get baseline vital signs at the time of admission.

➢ Temperature
Oral: 96.6 to 98.6 is normal.
Rectal: Would be one degree higher and most reliable.
Axillary (under the arm): Would be one degree lower and is the least reliable.

➢ Heart Rate (Pulse) and Respiration

Age	Normal heart rate (beats per minute)		Normal respiratory rate (breaths per minute)	
	Range	Typical example	Range	Typical example
Newborn	100–160	130	30–50	40
0–5 months	90–150	120	25–40	30
6–12 months	80–140	110	20–30	25
1–3 years	80–130	105	20–30	25
3–5 years	80–120	100	20–30	25
6–10 years	70–110	90	15–30	20
11–14 years	60–105	80	12–20	16
15–20 years	60–100	80	12–30	20

➢ Blood Pressure

Stage	Approximate age	Systolic		Diastolic	
		Range	Typical example	Range	Typical example
Infants	1 to 12 months	75-100	85	50–70	60
Toddlers	1 to 4 years	80-110	95	50–80	65
Preschoolers	3 to 5 years	80-110	95	50–80	65
School age	6 to 13 years	85-120	100	55–80	65
Adolescents	13 to 18 years	95-140	115	60–90	75

Temperature. There are a variety of thermometers; therefore, it is important to read the instructions provided by the manufacturer before using any type or brand of thermometers with clients. For the purpose of this training, the instructions listed below are generally for a digital oral thermometer.

    a. Be sure the client has not had anything to eat or drink for approximately 5 to 10 minutes prior to taking his or her temperature.
    b. Touch the client's forehead. Note the appearance and feel of the skin. For example, does the client's skin feel warm and moist, cold and clammy, or hot and dry?
    c. Place a clean sheath on the end of the thermometer that is to be placed in client's mouth.
    d. Turn thermometer on.
    e. Insert the thermometer into the client's mouth according to the manufacturer's instructions, which typically direct that it be inserted toward the back of the mouth under the tongue. Do not allow the client to bite the thermometer.
    f. After approximately 10 to 30 seconds, listen for the tone or beep, which signals a reading has been obtained.
    g. Record temperature reading.

    Other devices are available for measuring a client's:
        i.   armpit (axillary) temperature;
       ii.   rectal temperature;
      iii.   ear (aural) temperature;
      iv.   forehead (temporal artery) temperature.

Pulse. There are several locations on the body to assess a client's pulse. For this training, the underside of a client's wrist area along the radius bone will be used. The pulse is defined by the number of beats per minute.

    a. Place two or three fingertips (not the thumb) along the inside bone area on the underside of the wrist on the client's thumb side.
    b. Once the pulse is located, count the number of beats for 30 seconds.
    c. Multiply that number by two, which then equals the pulse.
    d. Make a written note of the pulse.
    e. If the pulse feels irregular (very fast, or weak, or seems to be skipping a beat) then take a full 60 seconds to assess the pulse and do not multiply that number by two.
    f. Make a written notation with the vital signs describing the unusual pulse rhythm or force.

Respirations. This is the number of breaths a client takes in one minute. Because clients may alter their breathing (consciously or unconsciously) when they realize their respirations are being counted, it is best to count their breaths when taking their temperature.

    a. Watch the client's chest rise and fall for 30 seconds.
    b. Multiply that number by two.
    c. Make a written note of the respirations.
    d. If the client's breathing is abnormal, count their breaths for a full 60 seconds and do not multiply that number by two.
    e. Make a written notation with the vital signs describing the unusual breathing. Note if the breathing is rapid, shallow, or labored. Note if the client is having trouble breathing and making unusual audible noises.

Blood Pressure. There are various blood pressure measuring devices available. Regardless of the type of blood pressure device, always read the manufacturer's directions for use. For the purpose of this training, the following steps are generally for electronic blood pressure measuring devices.

Steps for Obtaining Arm Blood Pressure

a. Direct the client to sit.
b. Ensure you have the correct cuff size for the specific client.
c. Wrap the blood pressure cuff around the client's left arm (preferred, not required) just above the elbow.
d. Press the start button on the blood pressure device.
e. Client should remain still and quiet.
f. Make a written notation of the blood pressure readings.
g. If an unusual blood pressure reading is obtained, either high or low, re-check blood pressure in 15 to 30 minutes.
h. Notify supervisor appropriate health care professional based upon the facility's policies and procedures when unusual blood pressure readings are obtained.

Steps for Obtaining Wrist Blood Pressure Reading

a. Direct the client to sit.
b. Place cuff on left wrist positioned according to manufacturer's directions.
c. Position client's left arm across his or her chest at approximately a 45 degree angle while having them cradle their left elbow with their right hand.
d. Press the start button on the blood pressure device.
e. If the wrist blood pressure measuring device does not start pumping or if an error reading is obtained, the client's left arm likely needs to be re-positioned to the correct angle of 45 degrees. When re-positioned correctly, the device should begin pumping and functioning properly.
f. Make a written notation of the blood pressure readings.
g. If an unusual blood pressure reading is obtained, either high or low, re-check blood pressure in 15 to 30 minutes.
h. Notify supervisor and/or an appropriately licensed medical care professional, based upon the facility's policies and procedures when unusual blood pressure readings are obtained.

When recording vital signs, the following abbreviations are acceptable.

T	–	temperature
P	–	pulse
R	–	respirations
BP	–	blood pressure

 Vital signs are recorded per facility policy and procedures. If any vital sign is not within normal limits, refer to the facility's policies and procedures for appropriate notification actions.

Section 14 - Storing and Disposing of Medications, & Maintaining an Inventory

Participants will be able to:
- understand how to store controlled medications versus other medications;
- understand how to dispose of medication per industry standards.

1. Storing and Securing Medication

   a. All medications must be stored in the original container in which they were dispensed by a licensed pharmacist and be maintained at an appropriate temperature. The labels must be legible. Do not make any changes to the labels.

   b. OTC medications must be kept in a locked cabinet/drawer. Controlled medications must be kept under a double lock, such as a locked cabinet inside a locked room.

   c. Keep refrigerated medication locked as well. This can mean a locked refrigerator, or a locked box inside a designated refrigerator. Refrigerated medications may not be stored with food. The refrigerator should be maintained thermostatically between 36° and 46°F (2° and 8°C).

   d. It is best practice to separate the daily scheduled medications from the "as needed" or prn medications.

2. Disposing of Medications

   a. Current and active prescriptions dispensed by a pharmacy for a specific client legally belong to that client. Therefore, when a client discharges from, or transitions out of a program, the legal guardian shall be given all of the client's medications that have been labeled by a pharmacy with client-specific information.

   b. All expired or discontinued medication shall be disposed of according to individual facility policies and procedures, by the appropriate means, and in compliance with applicable local, state and federal regulations. Medications must be destroyed beyond the possibility that they could be used again.

   At the time of this revision of the MATY curriculum, the Food and Drug Administration (FDA) and the Office of National Drug Control Policy (ONDCP) developed federal guidelines on drug disposal. Those guidelines are summarized below. However, when developing or reviewing facility policies and procedures, always check for new or updated laws and regulations through the Virginia Board of Pharmacy and Food and Drug Administration.
   - Virginia Board of Pharmacy at www.dhp.state.va.us/pharmacy.
   - Food and Drug Administration at www.fda.gov then type "drug disposal" in search window for listing of relevant guidelines and articles.

Federal Guidelines

1. Follow any specific disposal instructions on the prescription drug labeling or patient information that accompanies the medicine. Do not flush medicines down the sink or toilet unless this information specifically instructs you to do so*.

2. Take advantage of community drug take-back programs that allow the public to bring unused drugs to a central location for proper disposal. Call your city or county government's household trash and recycling service (see blue pages in phone book) to see if a take-back program is available in your community. The U.S. Drug Enforcement Administration, working with state and local law enforcement agencies, periodically sponsors National Prescription Drug Take-Back Days.

3. If no disposal instructions are given on the prescription drug labeling and no take-back program is available in your area, throw the drugs in the household trash following these steps. 1. Remove them from their original containers and mix them with an undesirable substance, such as used coffee grounds or kitty litter (this makes the drug less appealing to children and pets, and unrecognizable to people who may intentionally go through the trash seeking drugs). 2. Place the mixture in a sealable bag, empty can, or other container to prevent the drug from leaking or breaking out of a garbage bag.

See Appendix 7 for list of medicines recommended for disposal by flushing.

c. When destroying medications, the staff person's actions shall be witnessed by another staff person and documented. Documentation shall include the name of the staff person destroying the medications, the name of the witness, date, and the name and quantity of the medications.

3. Inventory of Medications

Controlled medications should be inventoried each day. Medication counts need to be documented per facility policy. Appendix 10 provides an example of a daily count form for controlled medications.

4. Dropped or Spilled Medication

 If a prescribed or OTC medication is dropped or spilt at any point during the administration process, the medication should be considered spoiled and disposed of according to your facility's policies and procedures for medication disposal.

Section 15 - Administering Eye Drops and Ointments

Participants will be able to:
- explain how to competently assist clients to administer eye drops and eye ointments;
- simulate how to assist clients to administer eye drops and eye ointments.

Eye Drops: When preparing eye drops, follow the steps below.

1. Ensure the physicians order has been transcribed to the individual's MAR.
2. Check the Six Rights.
3. Prepare supplies.
4. Wash hands.
5. Wear protective gloves if administering eye drops or ointments.
6. Never allow the tip of the dropper to touch any surface, including the eye.
7. Tilt the client's head back.
8. With index finger, gently pull client's lower eyelid downward away from eye to form pouch.
9. Drop medication in pouch.
10. Close the client's eye gently.
11. Instruct client to avoid blinking.
12. Instruct client to keep eye(s) closed for 1 to 2 minutes.
13. Discard gloves and wash hands.
14. Document in MAR.
15. Clean the medication administration area.

*Exception for treatment of glaucoma and/or inflammation – after placing drops in the client's eye(s), gently apply pressure to the inside corner of the eye to prevent drops from draining through the tear ducts.

Eye Ointment: When preparing eye ointment, follow the steps below.

1. Ensure the physicians order has been transcribed to the individual's MAR.
2. Check the Six Rights.
3. Prepare supplies.
4. Wash hands.
5. Wear protective gloves if administering eye drops or ointments.
6. Tilt the client's head back.
7. With index finger, gently pull client's lower eyelid downward away from eye to form pouch.
8. Without touching the tube to the client's eye(s), squeeze a thin strip of ointment into the inside margin of the lower eye lashes, about 1/3 of an inch.
9. Instruct client to keep eye(s) closed for 1 to 2 minutes.
10. Discard gloves and wash hands.
11. Document in MAR.
12. Clean the medication administration area.

Section 16 - Administering Ear Drops

Participants will be able to:
- explain how to competently assist clients to administer ear drops;
- simulate how to assist clients to administer ear drops.

When preparing ear drops, follow the steps below.

1. Ensure the physicians order has been transcribed to the individual's MAR.
2. Check the Six Rights.
3. Prepare supplies.
4. Wash hands.
5. Wear protective gloves.
6. Gently tilt the client's head so the ear being treated if facing up.
7. Using a clean tissue, wipe away any visible discharge from the outer ear only (never insert anything into the ear).
8. Gently pull ear lobe up and back to straighten ear canal.
9. Use dropper to administer medication into the ear canal without going past outer ear area.
10. Insert cotton ball into outer ear opening if necessary or ordered.
11. Have the client maintain the tilted head position with the treated ear facing upward for 5 minutes after the ear drops are administered. Consider having the client lay down.
12. Replace cap on medication.
13. Wash hands.
14. Document in MAR.
15. Clean the medication administration area.

Precautions

➢ Do not touch the dropper/applicator to any skin surface including the ear to help prevent contamination.

➢ Do not rinse dropper. May wipe tip of dropper with clean tissue and recap.

Section 17 - Administering Nasal Drops and Sprays

Participants will be able to:
- explain how to competently assist clients to administer nasal drops and sprays;
- simulate how to assist clients to administer nasal drops and sprays.

Nasal Drops: When preparing nasal drops, follow the steps below.

1. Ensure the physician's order has been transcribed to the individual's MAR.
2. Check the Six Rights.
3. Prepare supplies.
4. Wash hands.
5. Wear protective gloves.
6. Have client gently blow their nose.
7. Check dropper for cracks.
8. Gently tilt the client's head back while he or she is sitting or lying down. Nasal passageways should be near perpendicular to the floor.
9. Place drops in nostril. Aim the dropper along the back wall of the nostril, not straight up nostril opening.
10. Wipe dropper with clean tissue. Rinse dropper if there are visible signs or mucous or discharge.
11. Recap nasal drops container.
12. Wash hands.
13. Document in MAR.
14. Clean the medication administration area.

Nasal Sprays: When preparing nasal sprays, follow the steps below.

1. Ensure the physician's order has been transcribed to the individual's MAR.
2. Check the Six Rights.
3. Prepare supplies.
4. Wash hands.
5. Wear protective gloves.
6. Have client gently blow their nose.
7. Instruct client to sniff briskly while squeezing bottle quickly and firmly.
8. Spray once or twice in each nostril per prescriber's orders.
9. Wipe tip of spray bottle with clean tissue.
10. If nasal discharge is on bottle, rinse it with warm water then dry with tissue.
11. Recap tightly after use.
12. Wash hands.
13. Document in MAR.
14. Clean the medication administration area.

Note: Client may self-administer drops and spray once instructed if he/she can demonstrate competency. All Six Rights still apply to self-administered medications.

Section 18 - Administering Topical Medications

Participants will be able to:
- explain how to competently assist clients to administer topical medications;
- simulate how to assist clients to administer topical medications.

When preparing topical medications, follow the steps below.

1. Ensure the physician's order has been transcribed to the individual's MAR.
2. Check the Six Rights.
3. Prepare supplies.
4. Wash hands.
5. Wear protective gloves.
6. If indicated, shake medication.
7. Squeeze appropriate amount of medication into your gloved hand and/or medicine cup.
8. Apply to affected area. Start in the center and apply in a circular motion, taking care to not contaminate areas that have already been covered.
9. Do not cover with bandage unless directed by prescriber.
10. Do not apply topical medicine with bare fingers.
11. Do not apply directly from tube to the client's skin.
12. Recap medication.
13. Remove gloves and wash hands.
14. Document in MAR.
15. Clean the medication administration area.

Section 19 - Administering Compresses and Dressings

Participants will be able to:
- explain how to competently administer compresses and dressings;
- simulate how to administer compresses and dressings.

When administering compresses and dressings, follow the steps below.

1. Ensure the physician's order has been transcribed to the individual's MAR.
2. Check the Six Rights.
3. Prepare supplies.
4. Wash hands.
5. Wear protective gloves.
6. Prepare solution per prescriber's orders.
7. Soak the gauze in prepared solution and squeeze slightly.
8. Apply the compress to the affected area per prescriber's orders.
   a. Cold compress – keep cold by changing every 2 to 3 minutes or wrap in dry cloth over clothes and then apply ice bag. Check area frequently (every 20 minutes) for blueness or paleness.
   b. Warm compress – check temperature of the compress solution per prescriber's orders. Reheat compress by dipping into solution again. Check affected area frequently for redness and warmth.
9. Prevent compress from touching objects or persons to decrease the chance of passing germs.
10. Apply dressing per prescriber's orders.
11. Dispose of compress / dressing according to facility's procedures following Standard / Universal Precautions.
12. Remove gloves and wash hands.
13. Document in client's record or file (sometimes the prescriber will stipulate additional documentation in the MAR). Use the guidelines for documenting below.
14. Clean the medication administration area.

Guidelines for Documenting a Wound

1. Document the general appearance
   a. shape
   b. size – dime, nickel, quarter, approximate inches, etc.
   c. color – reddish, blue/green bruise, bright red, scab colored, etc.
   d. odor – describe if present
   e. same, better, or worse general appearance over period of minutes/hours/days

2. Document the signs of infection
   a. drainage – state if present/absent, include color description if present
   b. warmth – degree of warmth to the touch
   c. swelling – describe degree/size of swelling if present and changes over time
   d. discomfort – based on self-report, staff observations of client mobility, facial expression, rating on rating scale of 1 to 10 (10 = highest possible level of pain)
   e. discoloration of surrounding tissue

Section 20 - Administering Oral Hygiene Products

Participants will be able to:
- explain how to competently assist client to use oral hygiene products;
- simulate how to assist client to use oral hygiene products.

1. Examples of oral hygiene products
    a. OTC mouthwash
    b. prescription mouthwash
    c. toothpaste
    d. dental floss
    e. ointments or gels for mouth ulcers
    f. cavity fighting chewable tablets

2. Using oral hygiene products
    a. read and follow package label instructions
    b. read and follow pharmacy insert information
    c. refer to prescriber's instructions
    d. when administering gum ointment:
        i. gather and prepare supplies
        ii. check the Six Rights
        iii. wash hands
        iv. wear protective gloves
        v. if indicated, shake the medication
        vi. squeeze the amount of medication indicated onto the tip of a clean gloved finger
        vii. apply the medication evenly to the affected surface of the client's gum
        viii. if more medication is needed, use a different clean gloved finger tip
        ix. remove glove and wash hands
        x. document in MAR
        xi. clean the medication administration area

3. Dentists and dental hygienists routinely provide instructions and oral hygiene education to clients during appointments. It is recommended that programs specifically request hygiene education for their clients in the paperwork sent to the provider for the appointment.

Section 21 - Administering Transdermal Patches

Participants will be able to:
- explain how to competently assist client to administer transdermal patches;
- simulate how to assist client to use transdermal patches.

Transdermal patches are similar in appearance to band aids, first aid dressing, or medical tape. They are a means of delivering medication through skin. This means of delivery is chosen because clients may not be able to take pills, the medication needs to enter the body slowly, or in some cases because the client is uncooperative or unreliable in taking his or her medication. Examples of transdermal patches include birth control patches, nicotine patches to help a client stop smoking, and ADHD medication.

When administering transdermal patches, follow the steps below.

1. Ensure the physician's order has been transcribed to the individual's MAR.
2. Check the Six Rights.
3. Gather and prepare supplies.
4. Wash hands.
5. Wear protective gloves.
6. Remove old patch (if applicable) by folding in on itself.
7. Clean affected area of the skin as indicated by packaging instructions, pharmacy insert, or prescriber instructions.
8. Pat area dry with strong absorbent tissue.
9. Discard gloves and put on new protective gloves.
10. Carefully remove patch from packaging. Write the date and your initials on the new patch before application.
11. Apply the patch, often by peeling off backing to expose adhesive side of the patch, being careful to only touch the edges of the patch and not the middle portion.
12. Smooth patch onto skin and place gloved hand over patch for 10 seconds.
13. Check to be sure the patch is adhering properly.
14. Remove gloves.
15. Wash hands.
16. Document in MAR.
17. Clean and organize medication administration area.
18. If patch is a controlled medication, it must be disposed of in a sharps container.

Section 22 - Administering Soaks and Sitz Baths

Participants will be able to:
- explain how to competently administer soaks and sitz baths;
- simulate how to administer soaks and sitz baths.

A sitz bath is a special bath basin and solution to treat problems in the rectal area such as hemorrhoids.

When administering a sitz bath, follow the steps below.

1. Ensure the physician's order has been transcribed to the individual's MAR.
2. Check the Six Rights.
3. Prepare supplies.
4. Wash hands.
5. Wear protective gloves if area infected or bloody.
6. Place client in comfortable position.
7. Prepare solution per prescriber's orders.
8. Maintain proper temperature for soaking solution or sitz bath throughout treatment.
9. Soak limb and/or maintain sitz bath for prescribed time.
10. Maintain clean conditions.
11. Remove gloves and wash hands.
12. Document in MAR.
13. Clean the medication administration area.

 Please checks your facility policy for the administration and supervision for administering soaks and sitz baths.

Section 23 - Administering Rectal Suppositories

Participants will be able to:
- explain how to competently assist client to administer rectal suppositories;
- simulate how to assist client to use rectal suppositories.

Rectal suppositories are used to treat various conditions such as hemorrhoids, constipation, severe nausea, or vomiting. For a client with a seizure disorder, a suppository might be the fastest acting route of medication administration. The suppository is a wax-like substance that can melt quickly after insertion.

When administering rectal suppositories, follow the steps below.

1. Ensure the physician's order has been transcribed to the individual's MAR.
2. Check the Six Rights.
3. Prepare supplies.
4. Wash hands.
5. Wear protective gloves.
6. Suppositories should be stored in cool temperature. If suppository is too soft, place briefly in refrigerator or run under cold water before removing the wrapper.
7. Remove the foil wrapper.
8. Moisten suppository with water or KY jelly for easier insertion.
9. Have client lie on left side with right leg flexed up.
10. Push suppository well up into rectum with finger up to the second knuckle of the finger.
11. Remove gloves.
12. Wash hands.
13. Document in MAR.
14. Clean and organize medication administration area.

 Check your facility policy for the administration and supervision for administering rectal suppositories.

Section 24 - Administering Vaginal Products

Participants will be able to:
- explain how to competently assist client to administer vaginal products;
- simulate how to assist client to use vaginal products.

Vaginal products are used to treat conditions such as yeast infections or other gynecological problems.

When administering vaginal products, follow the steps below.

1. Ensure the physician's order has been transcribed to the individual's MAR.
2. Check the Six Rights
3. Prepare supplies
4. Wash hands
5. Wear protective gloves
6. Follow packaging instructions, pharmacy insert, or prescriber instructions to prepare
7. Prepare vaginal cream/ointment using special applicator supplied with product
8. *Client should lie on back with knees drawn up
9. Using applicator, insert medication into vagina as far can be done without using force
10. Release medicine by pushing plunger
11. Wash applicator with hot, soapy water if it needs to be used again
12. Remove gloves
13. Wash hands
14. Document in MAR
15. Clean and organize medication administration area

*Optional – client may stand and place one foot on edge of bathtub, chair, etc. and insert applicator into vagina. Check product instructions or insert as to whether the client should be directed to lie down for 30 minutes after medication insertion.

 Check your facility policy for the administration and supervision for administering vaginal products.

Section 25 - Asthma

Participants will be able to:
- accurately list asthma episode triggers and early warning signs;
- accurately describe prevention measures;
- describe key elements of an Asthma Awareness Information Sheet for child and adolescent clients;
- explain and demonstrate how to competently assist clients to use asthma inhaler products.

Asthma is a long-term physical disorder of the lungs' airways in which breathing becomes difficult and labored. During an asthma episode, airways become inflamed and therefore smaller in reaction to environmental triggers (allergens such as dust, pollen, or pet dander). Asthma episodes may also be the result of genetic factors, physical activity, or stress.

One general asthma condition is chronic or steady-state asthma in which persons experience some ongoing tightness in the chest, throat clearing, a night time cough, or shortness of breath. Long-acting medications, monitoring, and healthy lifestyle changes are the typical approaches to management of this category of asthma.

The second major asthma condition is a sudden worsening of symptoms, an asthma attack or acute episode, in which breathing becomes difficult, there is tightness in the chest and possible wheezing. Fast acting medications are necessary to help clients with this type of asthma condition.

For current best practices and form templates, reference the American Academy of Allergy, Asthma, and Immunology (www.aaaai.org).

See Appendix 5 for a sample of an Asthma Awareness Information Sheet.

ASTHMA FACTS

TRIGGERS: Irritants, allergens, or emotions such as high anxiety can start an asthma episode. Every client with asthma will have his or her own unique triggers.

• Dust	• Illnesses such as respiratory infections, cold, or flu
• Pollen	• Exercise
• Mold	• Cold air / humidity
• Perfume	• Emotions such as excitement or anxiety
• Pet dander	• Tobacco smoke

PREVENTIVE MEASURES: Actions that can decrease the number or severity or asthma episodes.

• Don't use perfumes or other strongly scented products	• Control dust, pollens, molds, allergens, and irritants in child care areas
• Keep pets out of child care areas at all times	• Limit outdoor activities when pollen or air pollution levels are high
• Prohibit all smoking	• Use medication as directed
• Avoid asthma triggers	

EARLY WARNING SIGNS: Mild symptoms usually occur <u>before</u> an asthma episode. The ability to recognize early warning signs is helpful because staff and clients can take quick action. Early action may decrease the seriousness of the attack or even prevent an asthma episode from occurring. Each client with asthma will have his or her own unique early warning signs.

• Behavior changes such as nervousness	• Headache
• Rapid breathing	• Fatigue
• Wheezing, coughing	• Changes in peak flow meter readings
• Stuffy or runny nose	• Watery eyes, itchy throat, or chin

SIGNS AND SYMPTOMS OF AN ASTHMA EPISODE: If a staff person notices the client experiencing any of the following symptoms, he or she should take action immediately as indicated in the client's asthma action care plan.

• Acting agitated or scared	• Breathing with lips pursed
• Breathing rapidly	• Sitting with shoulders hunched over
• Wheezing	• Is unusually pale
• Having a persistent cough	• Having trouble breathing when lying down

TREATMENT OPTIONS FOR CLIENTS WITH ASTHMA

Medication Used to Treat Asthma

Many clients with asthma need to take medication. There are two types of asthma medication that children and adolescents can be prescribed.

- **Long-acting medication.** Some clients may need to take medication on a regular basis, usually daily, to prevent an asthma episode. These medications are sometimes called controller medications. Examples of this category of medications include Advair Diskus and Singulair.

- **Fast-acting medication.** Some clients may only take medication when they are experiencing an asthma episode. These medications work quickly to relieve asthma symptoms. They are sometimes called reliever or rescue medications. Albuterol is one common example of this type of medication.

Some clients with asthma may need to take a combination of long-acting and fast-acting medication to keep their asthma under control.

Medication Delivery Systems

Clients can be given asthma medication in many forms such as oral tablets, metered dose inhalers, inhalers using a spacer device, dry powder inhalers, and liquid medication for nebulizer use. The form of medication the client receives may be dependent on the type of medication and the age of the child or adolescent.

- **Oral Medication.** Oral medications are easy for many clients to take. Some asthma medications are available as oral tablets and chewable medication.

- **Metered Dose Inhaler.** A metered dose inhaler is used to deliver medication directly to the client's lungs. To get the desired effect of the medication, the client must be able to properly use the inhaler. Clients as young as age five can be taught to properly use an inhaler.

- **Meter Dose Inhaler with a Spacer Device.** A metered dose inhaler can often be attached to a spacer device. The spacer device holds the medicine in a chamber allowing the client to breathe in the medicine over several breaths. The use of a spacer device with an inhaler allows a younger child (3-5 years of age) to use an inhaler successfully.

- **Dry Powder Inhaler.** A dry powder inhaler is used to deliver dry powder medication directly to the lungs. Dry powder inhalers work differently than metered-dose inhalers; the inhaler is activated when the client takes a breath. Always follow the manufacturer's directions for use and care if a client in your facility uses a dry powder inhaler.

- **Nebulizer Machines.** A nebulizer machine converts liquid medicine into a mist that can be breathed into the lungs. No special breathing techniques are necessary when using a nebulizer. This allows very young clients to get needed medicine into the lungs. Because children do not need to follow any special breathing techniques, children under 5-years-old are often prescribed medication using a nebulizer machine.

Managing Asthma

Clients that have moderate or severe asthma often need to keep track of how well their asthma is controlled. Children over three years old can often be taught to use a peak flow meter to do this.

- **Peak Flow Meter.** A peak flow meter is a portable, hand-held device used to measure how hard and fast a client can push air out of his lungs. Each time the client uses the peak flow meter, he or she gets a measurement or a reading. Measurements with a peak flow meter help the client's parent and staff person monitor the asthma. These measurements can be important in helping the client's prescriber select medicines to keep asthma under control.

SAMPLE ASTHMA AWARENESS INFORMATION SHEET

Client's Name: _____ **Date of Birth:** _____
Parent(s) or Guardian(s) Name: _____
Emergency phone numbers: Mother _____ Father _____

Primary health care provider's name: _____ **Phone:** _____
Current asthma medication: _____

Known triggers for this client's asthma (circle all that apply):

colds	mold	exercise	tree pollens
dust	strong odors	grass	flowers
excitement	weather changes	animals	smoke

foods (specify): _____
other (specify): _____

Activities for which this client has needed special attention in the past (circle all that apply)

OUTDOORS	INDOORS
Field trip to see animals	Painting or renovations
Running hard	Art projects with chalk, glue
Gardening	Pet care
Outdoor on cold or windy days	Recent pesticide application
Playing in freshly cut grass	Sitting on carpets

Others (specify): _____

Typical signs and symptoms of the client's asthma episodes (circle all that apply):

Fatigue	Breathing faster	Dark circles under eyes
Flaring nostrils	Persistent coughing	Gray or blue lips or fingernails
Difficulty playing	Difficulty eating	Difficulty drinking
Difficulty talking	Face red, pale or swollen	Wheezing
Sucking in chest/neck	Mouth open (panting)	Agitation
Grunting	Restlessness	Complains of chest pain or tightness

Others (specify): _____

Remember to always bring fast-acting asthma medication with the client during off-site activities. If severe sudden asthma problem persists or worsens after fast-acting medication is administered as prescribed, seek emergency medical assistance.

Parent/Guardian Signature: _____ Date: _____

INHALED MEDICATION ADMINISTRATION
ORAL METERED DOSE INHALER

- **PREPARATION PHASE**

  1. Remove the inhaler from the box and compare it against the container.
  2. Check the Six Rights.
  3. Wash hands.
  4. If indicated, shake the medication.
  5. Put on protective gloves.
  6. If the client is able, have him or her stand.
  7. Remove the cap from the inhaler.
  8. Hold the inhaler between index finger and thumb.

- **ADMINISTRATION PHASE**

  1. Ask child to breathe out.
  2. Have the child put the inhaler mouthpiece into his or her mouth and close his or her lips loosely around it.
  3. With the client's head titled slightly back, ask him or her to take in a slow deep breath.
  4. As the client does this, press down on the inhaler canister to release the spray.
  5. Have the client hold his or her breath for a few seconds then exhale with lips pursed.
  6. If additional puffs are needed or prescribed, wait the recommended time before giving the second puff or at least one minute.
  7. Wipe off the inhaler mouthpiece with a clean tissue and replace the cap.
  8. Remove gloves and discard using the appropriate technique.
  9. Wash hands.
  10. Document in MAR.
  11. Clean and organize medication administration area.

- **CLEANING A METERED DOSE INHALER AFTER EACH USE**

  1. Remove the medication canister from the mouthpiece.
  2. Take off the inhaler cap.
  3. Rinse both the mouthpiece and the cap under warm running water for a minute. Never put the canister of medication in the water.
  4. Shake off the excess water.
  5. Allow the parts to air dry on a clean towel or wipe with a lint free towel then reassemble.

INHALED MEDICATION ADMINISTATION
ORAL METERED DOSE INHALER WITH SPACER

A spacer is a chamber or tube like device that attaches to a pressurized inhaler to slow down the delivery of medication. The spacer allows more medication to reach the lungs by decreasing the amount of medication that gets deposited in the mouth or the throat area.

- **PREPARATION PHASE**

  1. Remove the inhaler from the box and compare it against the container.
  2. Check the Six Rights.
  3. Wash hands.
  4. Put on protective gloves.
  5. Shake the medication if indicated.
  6. Take the cap off the inhaler mouthpiece and attach the inhaler to the client's spacer. If a mask is needed, attach the client's mask to the spacer.

- **ADMINISTRATION PHASE**

  1. Have the client stand.
  2. Have the client insert the spacer mouthpiece into his or her mouth and close his or her lips loosely around it. If a mask is attached to the spacer, place the mask on the client's face covering both the nose and mouth.
  3. With the client's head tilted slightly back, ask him or her to take a slow deep breath. As the client does this, press down on the inhaler to release the spray into the spacer.
  4. Have the client inhale deeply and slowly over 3-5 seconds.
  5. Keeping the spacer mouthpiece in the client's mouth, have him or her hold their breath for a few seconds then breathe out into the spacer.
  6. With the spacer mouthpiece still in the client's mouth, have him or her continue breathing in and out into the spacer for at least three more cycles to be sure all the medication in the spacer chamber is used.
  7. If additional puffs are needed, wait the recommended time per the health care provider's instructions before giving the second puff.
  8. Take the spacer off the inhaler, wipe the spacer mouthpiece with a tissue, and replace the cap.
  9. Take off gloves and discard in an appropriate manner.
  10. Wash hands.
  11. Document in MAR.
  12. Clean and organize medication administration area.

- **CLEANING A METERED DOSE INHALER AFTER EACH USE**

  1. See instructions for metered dose inhaler from previous page.
  2. Clean spacer as directed by the manufacturer.

INHALED MEDICATION ADMINISTRATION
USING A NEBULIZER

A nebulizer is a device used to administer asthma medication. It has an electrically powered compressor that forces air through the device to produce a fine medication mist that is inhaled through a mask or mouthpiece.

It is important to note that the steps for each nebulizer set-up and administration are different based on the type of nebulizer machine used. Always follow the manufacturer's instructions when giving a nebulizer treatment.

The following are general principles for giving a nebulizer treatment to a client regardless of machine type.

- **PREPARATION PHASE**

  1. Check the Six Rights.
  2. Check to make sure all of the necessary nebulizer parts to administer the medication are present.
  3. Plug the nebulizer compressor into a power source.
  4. Turn on the machine to make sure it is working. Turn the machine off again.
  5. Put on protective gloves.
  6. Attach the tubing and nebulizer parts to the compressor.
  7. Remove the medication/vial and compare it to the medication container.
  8. Pour the prescribed amount of medication into the nebulizer medication cup. If the medicine needs to be diluted, carefully follow the health care provider instructions on how to dilute the medication.

- **ADMINISTRATION PHASE**

  1. Turn on the nebulizer machine.
  2. Make sure there is a mist coming out of the mouthpiece before placing it into the client's mouth or placing the mask over the client's nose and mouth.
  3. Place the mouthpiece in the client's mouth or place the mask over the client's nose and mouth.
  4. Have the client breathe normally while remaining seated in upright position.
  5. The treatment is done when no more liquid is in the medication cup.
  6. Take off gloves and discard in an appropriate manner.
  7. Wash hands.
  8. Document in MAR.
  9. Clean and organize medication administration area.

CARE OF A NEBULIZER MACHINE

Nebulizer machines and parts require special care and cleaning to reduce the risk of harmful bacterial growth. Below are general principles for caring for a nebulizer machine. The steps may vary based on the type of nebulizer machine being used. Always follow the manufacturer's instructions when cleaning a nebulizer machine and when to change the machine filters.

- **AFTER EACH USE**

    1. Disconnect the nebulizer parts (mask or mouthpiece and the medicine cup) from the tubing.
    2. If condensation is present inside the tubing, run the machine for 10-20 seconds to dry the inside of the tubing.
    3. Disconnect the tubing from the nebulizer and place it in a sealable plastic bag.
    4. The tubing should never be rinsed or put in water.
    5. Wash the remaining nebulizer parts with a mild dishwashing soap and warm water.
    6. Rinse the nebulizer parts under a strong stream of warm running water for at least 30 seconds. If possible, use distilled or sterile water as a final rinse.
    7. Shake off any excess water.
    8. Allow the nebulizer parts to air dry on a clean cloth or paper towel. The parts may be dried with a lint free towel.
    9. Once dry, place the remaining nebulizer parts into the sealable plastic along with the tubing.

- **SHARING OF NEBULIZER MACHINES**

    It is acceptable practice to share a nebulizer compressor machine between two or more clients unless the nebulizer air compressor is labeled "for single patient use".

    If you are sharing a nebulizer compressor machine, each child must have his or her own tubing, medication cup, and mouthpiece or facemask. In addition, the manufacturer's instructions regarding use and care of the machine must be followed.

Section 26 – Administering an Epinephrine Autoinjector

Participants will be able to:
- explain how to competently use and inject an epinephrine autoinector;
- simulate how to use the auto-injector device.

An epinephrine autoinjector, commonly referred to as an EpiPen (a specific brand), is used in an emergency situation when an allergic client is exposed to an allergen that results in a severe allergic reaction or anaphylactic shock. Anaphylactic shock consists of a sudden drop in blood pressure and extreme difficulty in breathing and can result in death. Clients can have severe allergic reactions to bee stings, peanuts, shellfish, and latex, for example.

For clients known or suspected to have a strong allergic reaction or anaphylactic risk, remember to always bring at least one epinephrine autoinjector dose to off-site activities and have it readily available. Remember to check the expiration date regularly.

Different brands of epinephrine autoinjectors may require different administration procedures. Follow your facility's specific policies and procedures for administration pursuant to the different brands. The following instructions are specific to the EpiPen brand.

1. Remove epinephrine autoinjector from protective package or tube.
2. Grasp the unit with the black or orange tip pointing toward the thigh. Form a fist around the unit.
3. With the other hand, pull off the gray safety cap or release. (Do not remove gray safety release until ready to use.)
4. Hold epinephrine autoinjector firmly with the black tip near the outer thigh. Never place thumb, fingers or hand over the black tip.
5. Swing and jab the epinephrine autoinjector firmly into the outer thigh for approximately 10 seconds. (Count to 10.)
6. The injection is then complete. Remove the epinephrine autoinjector from the thigh.
7. Massage the injection area for 10 seconds.
8. Call 911 for emergency services and support.
9. Sometimes a second injection may be necessary, but always consult a licensed medical care provider before administering a second dose.
10. Dispose of the epinephrine autoinjector appropriately in a sharps container.

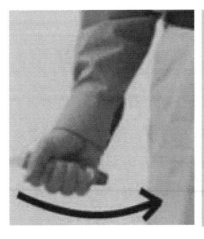 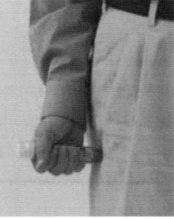 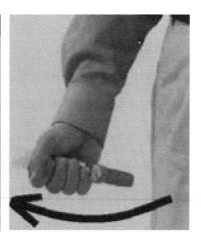

Section 27 – Diabetes

Participants will be able to:
- define what diabetes is as a medical condition;
- define Type I and Type II diabetes;
- list symptoms of diabetes and warning signs;
- describe treatments, interventions, and recommended lifestyle behaviors to manage diabetes.

This section is intended as an overview of diabetes and diabetes management. To appropriately care for clients with diabetes, specific instructions from the client's health care provider are required, which would be the standard and best practice if the client lived at home or attended a public school. Additional information can be found at www.diabetes.org, the American Diabetes Association, and www.virginiadiabetescouncil.org.

Definition and Description of Diabetes

Diabetes Type 1 / Insulin Dependent is a metabolic disorder that leads to persistent hyperglycemia, which is abnormally high sugar in the blood.

Glucose is the sugar molecule that is the body's fuel used for energy. It can be stored as fat or stored in the liver to be used at a later time.

In a healthy individual, food is eaten and starches, sugars, and proteins are eventually broken down into sugar. The sugar enters the blood stream and then insulin, reacting to the fluctuation in blood sugar, is secreted by the pancreas to carry it into the cells. The sugar in the cells is then used for energy.

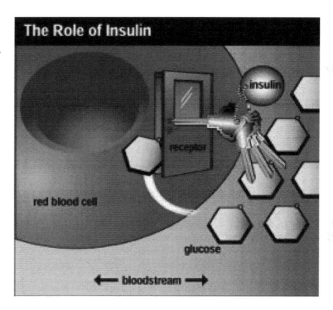

If there is not enough insulin, or the insulin is not able to carry sugar into the cells, it stays in the blood stream and this is the condition called diabetes. If untreated, this can lead to many serious complications and death. Diabetes can affect the immune system so that the body cannot fight infection. Other problems include nerve cell damage, kidney damage, eye problems, and heart disease. There is no cure for diabetes, but it can be controlled to decrease these risk factors.

The Diabetes Medical Management Plan (DMMP) is comonly used by health care providers to manage clients' diabetes. The American Diabetes Association has a sample DMMP available for viewing and downloading on their website at www.diabetes.org. (search for "DMMP").

<u>Types of Diabetes</u>: There are two types of diabetes.

Type I Diabetes (Insulin Dependent)

- ➢ Can occur at any age, but usually between 8 and 12 years.
- ➢ Little or no insulin is produced, so insulin injections are required.
- ➢ May be caused by a virus that destroys cells in the pancreas.
- ➢ Onset is abrupt and dramatic.

Signs & Symptoms of Type I Diabetes

- ➢ excessive urination
- ➢ excessive thirst
- ➢ dramatic weight loss
- ➢ weakness
- ➢ irritability
- ➢ if untreated, it rapidly progresses into acidosis and finally coma

Type II Diabetes (Non-Insulin Dependent)

- ➢ Usually occurs after age 40, but can occur at any time.
- ➢ The body still makes some insulin, but it is not enough or it cannot work properly.
- ➢ Can be treated with diet and exercise, oral medications and/or with insulin.
- ➢ Causes:
  - o Obesity
  - o Family history
  - o Stress
  - o Illness or injury

Signs and Symptoms of Type II Diabetes

- ➢ increased urination and thirst
- ➢ hunger
- ➢ feeling tired
- ➢ frequent infections
- ➢ blurred vision
- ➢ slow healing sores or cuts

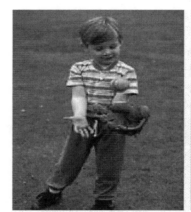 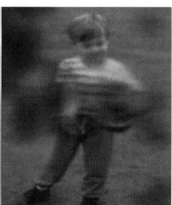

Normal vision   Vision with diabetic retinopathy

<u>Treatment Goals</u>

The goal of the client with diabetes is to maintain blood sugar at consistently normal levels to avoid complications. Every person is different so every treatment plan will be different. The prescriber will diagnose the client and give him or her a plan to follow. The client with diabetes needs to have a healthy balance of diet, exercise, and oral medications/insulin. The client with diabetes needs to have a structured and consistent life routine.

Diet and Exercise

Diet and exercise are important for every client with diabetes. Regular meals and a variety of foods are critical. Three meals a day with one or two snacks are often advised. Clients should avoid foods high in sugar and fat, and a well balanced diet should be followed. The challenge for the client is to eat varied foods yet similar amounts of food on a daily basis. A variety of foods, along with maintaining good glucose control, is necessary for normal growth and development.

Carbohydrates have the greatest effect on blood sugar. The Create Your Plate guide is a basic guide to choosing healthy food. Visit the American Diabetes Association (http://www.diabetes.org/food-and-fitness/food/planning-meals/create-your-plate/) and the National Diabetes Information Clearinghouse (http://diabetes.niddk.nih.gov/) for more information and resources.

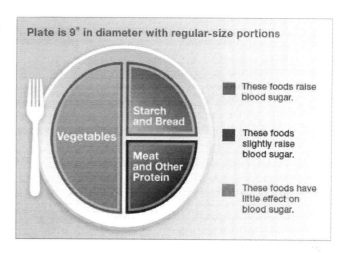

Clients with diabetes should exercise every day. It is more important and healthy for a client with diabetes to exercise 10 to 20 minutes daily compared to 1 hour a week. The muscles use energy during exercise, and therefore exercise lowers the blood sugar.

Snacks and meals are often a mixture of carbohydrates, protein and fat. Carbohydrates are broken down into sugar faster than protein or fat. Foods high in carbohydrates are breads, pasta, grains, fruits, milk and sugars. Meats and most vegetables are low in carbohydrates. Foods are assigned a number that represents a number of carbohydrates. If it can be determined how many carbohydrates are ingested, the amount of insulin a client needs can be determined, programmed into an insulin pump and delivered. (Insulin pumps are described later in this section.)

Monitoring Blood Glucose

There are many monitors from which a client can choose. The prescriber will recommend the monitor that best suits the client's needs. Blood glucose testing gives a client an immediate reading for their current blood glucose. Everyone has a different regimen, from testing several times a day to a few times a week. It depends upon how well controlled a client's diabetic condition can be with treatment. Soon after the diagnosis of diabetes, it is important for clients to check their glucose levels frequently because it helps them learn how different foods affect their condition. If clients are insulin dependent, they often check their glucose before breakfast, lunch, dinner, and at bedtime. Additional checks are needed if the client is sick because food intake may change during those times and during sickness in general. Adjustments may be needed for the insulin during those times.

Sample of Daily Record of Insulin Injections

Date	Time	Amount of Insulin	Blood Glucose Level	Injection Site

A record of all glucose readings and insulin injections should be kept along with how the client feels. If the glucose level is high, the client should make notes of what was eaten that may account for the high reading. A history of the glucose readings will usually be recorded and stored in the glucometer. This information may be tracked in the client's MAR. A sample form for recording insulin injections can be found in Appendix 9.

Testing Blood Glucose

1. Gather supplies.
   a. Lancet
   b. Injector
   c. Glucometer
   d. Strip
2. Wash hands.
3. Put on protective gloves
4. Dangle arm to increase blood flow and choose a finger to stick.
5. Remove injector top and put lancet in the injector.
6. Place top back on the injector.
7. Set the injector and place it firmly against the side of a finger. Do not place it on the pads of the finger where there are more nerve endings.
8. Press the trigger to release the lancet.
9. Put some pressure near the injected spot.
10. Place a drop of blood on the strip.
11. Wait for the reading.

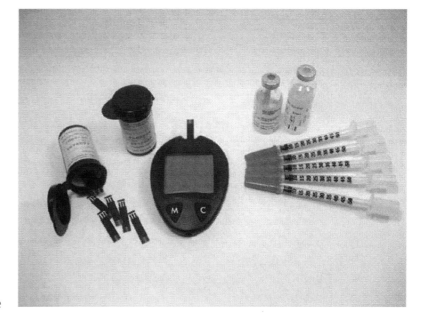

Insulin

There are a variety of insulins. They differ in how quickly they work, how long they work, and when they peak. Common insulin formulations include:

- **Humalog:** fast acting in 5 minutes, peaking in 1 hour, and complete in 3 hours
- **Humulin R (Regular):** short acting, takes 30 minutes to act, peaks in 3 hours, and is complete in 6 to 8 hours
- **Humulin N (NPH):** intermediate acting, takes 2 hours to act, and continues for 10 to 12 hours
- **Lantus** is long acting. Onset is 1-2 hours and can last 24 hours without a specific peak time
- **Pre-Mixed Insulin:** common pre-mixed insulins are Regular, NPH and fast acting. Pre-mix insulin comes in glass bottles. The client should always have an extra bottle in case one is broken. The bottles should be stored in a refrigerator. If unopened, it is good until the expiration date. If opened or unopened, it can stay out of the refrigerator for 28 days, but then should be discarded.

Please reference American Diabetes Association for current insulin formulations and their actions pertaining to clients at your facility.

Handling Insulin

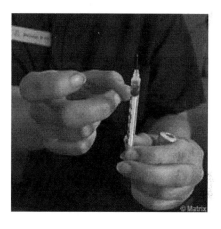

Gather supplies: insulin bottles
proper insulin syringe
alcohol swab
cotton

Insulin Administration Procedures

1. Wash hands.
2. Remove bottle from refrigerator.
3. If a new bottle, take the dust cover off and clean the rubber with an alcohol swab.
4. Gently roll the insulin bottle between your hands to mix it without causing bubbles.
5. Insulin is measured in units and requires an insulin syringe to be used.

Insulin syringes measure up to 50 units or 100 units. **Be Careful** to note if the lines on the syringe represent 1 unit (as on the 30 and 50 unit syringes) or 2 units (as on the 100 unit syringe). Choose the syringe that you need.

6. Put protective gloves on.
7. Remove the cap of the syringe and pull the plunger down, drawing in air to the line of the required number of units.
8. Insert the needle into the rubber top of the bottle and inject the air into the bottle. This is to replace the amount of insulin being removed from the bottle so that a vacuum is not created in the bottle.
9. Turn the bottle upside down and slowly pull the plunger down. There is air in the bore of the needle, so there will some air bubbles.

10. Draw the syringe past the line of the amount needed and tap the syringe to get bubbles to float up.
11. Then push the plunger up so the air bubbles go into the vial. This may be repeated as necessary. Make sure there are no bubbles as they replace needed insulin.
12. Then draw back the plunger so the top of the plunger is exactly at the line of what is needed for that dose of insulin.

Injecting the insulin

13. Choose an injection site. See diagram. It is important to rotate sites because if a site is repeatedly used, scar tissue will develop which will slow the absorption of the insulin.
14. Make sure site is clean.
15. Pinch up the skin.
16. Push the needle into the skin at a 90 degree angle.
17. Push the plunger all the way to the needle.
18. Wait a few seconds then withdraw the needle.
19. Do not rub the area.
20. Dispose of the syringe in a sharps box.
21. Do not recap the needle.
22. Make a note of where the injection was made.

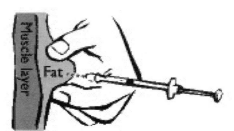

Pinching the skin to give an insulin injection. A small pinch with the finger and thumb is enough.

Preparing a Mixed Dose of Insulin

Sometimes a combination of insulins may be mixed in one syringe so that only one injection is required. Often the morning dose includes a mixture of fast acting and intermediate acting insulin. This mix will cover breakfast and lunch.

1. Check the Six Rights.
2. Determine the amount of insulin needed.
3. Get both bottles and rotate them gently between your hands.
4. The short acting (Regular or R) needs to be drawn up before the intermediate (NPH or N). To help remember this, you may think clear before cloudy. The R is clear, and the N is cloudy. Put the amount of air to displace the insulin in the intermediate bottle first.
5. For example, 8 units of R and 6 units of NPH may be needed.
6. Get 6 units of air and inject it into the NPH insulin first.
7. Get 8 units of air and inject it into the R (regular) insulin and withdraw the insulin. There may be bubbles because air is in the bore of the needle.
8. You may tap the syringe to get the bubbles to rise to the top of the syringe and push them out with the plunger.
9. Get the exact amount of insulin needed.
10. Then put the same syringe into the bottle of the intermediate acting insulin. (Air has already been injected into this bottle in a previous step.)
11. 8 units of regular has already been drawn, now draw it up to 14. This is the total of both insulins.
12. Then proceed to inject.

Injection Site Rotation

Typically, a prescriber or nurse specialist will help clients to establish an insulin injection routine and rotation. Information provided by those healthcare professionals is useful to staff working with clients with diabetes.

Insulin is injected into the fat, not the muscle, to be absorbed best.

There are four sites that can be injected:
1. Abdomen
2. Arms
3. Legs
4. Buttocks

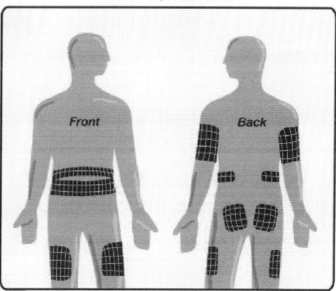

Insulin injection areas

The insulin is most rapidly absorbed in the abdomen. The sites should be rotated. If the same site is used consistently, the absorption rate will be slowed down. Keep track of where the injections are given so as not to overuse a particular area of the body.

See Appendix 9 for a sample tracking form of insulin injections.

One example of a common rotation site schedule is listed below.

1. Abdomen (stomach area)
    a. upper abdomen then lower abdomen
    b. right abdomen area then left abdomen area

2. Thigh
    a. right thigh upper area then lower area
    b. left thigh upper area then lower area

Insulin Pens and Pumps

When diet and exercise cannot control blood sugars, oral medications or insulin may be used. The only way insulin can be administered is through an injection. There are three methods for delivering an injection.

1. Single syringe dose (as described above)
2. Insulin pen
3. Insulin pump

Each method injects insulin into subcutaneous tissue. The insulin pen is prefilled with multiple doses. The needed amount is dialed on the pen and delivered, and then the needle is changed for the next dose.

An insulin pump is approximately the same size as a pager or cell phone that can be attached to a client's belt or clothing. Soft tubing connects the pump to a small cannula (stiff but flexible tubing designed to deliver or remove fluid from just under the skin). The tubing and cannula are taped into place for one to two days at a time to deliver insulin. The pump can be programmed to meet the needs of the individual client. For instance, the pump can be set to deliver a continuous basal rate (continuous and typically low supply of insulin), and when a meal is consumed, it can be programmed to deliver an additional dose of insulin to compensate for the meal. The amount of insulin is calculated by counting carbohydrates according to doctor's orders or the DMMP (Diabetes Medication Management Plan).

Adverse Reactions to Insulin

Adverse reactions to insulin can range from redness and itching at the injection site to more severe symptoms, such as difficulty breathing and increased heart rate. Hypoglycemia (low blood sugar described below) can result from too much insulin or not enough food. Onset of hypoglycemia can be sudden and result in insulin shock, which is an emergency situation. Glucose (i.e., sugar) would need to be administered in this situation.

Procedures for Low Blood Sugar (Hypoglycemia)

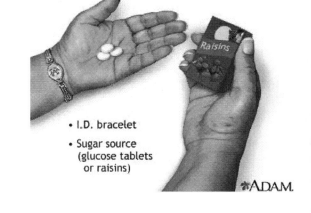

- I.D. bracelet
- Sugar source (glucose tablets or raisins)

Causes: too little food, or skipped meal
too much insulin or diabetic medicine
more active than usual, extra exercise

Onset: sudden, may progress to insulin shock

Symptoms: feeling shaky   fast heartbeat
sweating   dizziness
feeling anxious   hunger
blurred vision   weakness or fatigue
headache   irritable

Treatment:
- Call 911 or emergency services if the client loses consciousness.

- Per doctor's orders and/or DMMP. For clients at risk of severe hypoglycemia, glucagon may be prescribed according to the client's DMMP.

- Give something that can be absorbed quickly to elevate the blood sugar - orange juice, raisins, or a regular soda.

- Glucose tablets.

- Wait a few minutes and take the blood sugar level again.

- Do not give a sandwich at this time because it will slow down the absorption of needed fluid in the stomach, and therefore delay the process of the sugar getting into the blood.

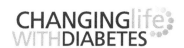
Hypoglycemia (Low Blood Glucose)

Some Symptoms:

Causes: Too little food or skipping a meal; too much insulin or diabetes pills; more active than usual.

Onset: Often sudden.

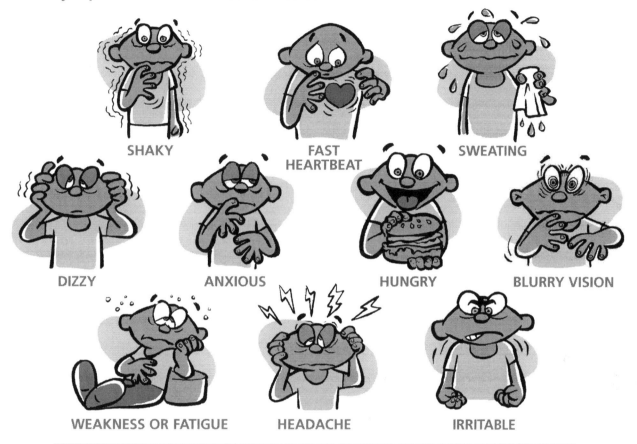

SHAKY

FAST HEARTBEAT

SWEATING

DIZZY

ANXIOUS

HUNGRY

BLURRY VISION

WEAKNESS OR FATIGUE

HEADACHE

IRRITABLE

IF LOW BLOOD GLUCOSE IS LEFT UNTREATED, YOU MAY PASS OUT AND NEED MEDICAL HELP.

What Can You Do?

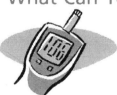

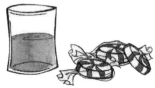

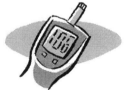

CHECK your blood glucose, right away. If you can't check, treat anyway.

TREAT by eating 3 to 4 glucose tablets or 3 to 5 hard candies you can chew quickly (such as peppermints), or by drinking 4-ounces of fruit juice, or 1/2 can of regular soda pop.

CHECK your blood glucose again after 15 minutes. If it is still low, treat again. If symptoms don't stop, call your healthcare provider.

For more information, call the Novo Nordisk Tip Line at
1-800-260-3730 or visit us online at ChangingDiabetes-us.com.

© Novo Nordisk Inc.   126379R   ChangingDiabetes-us.com   6/2006

novo nordisk®

Procedures for High Blood Sugar (Hyperglycemia)

Causes: too much food
not enough insulin or oral medication
illness
stress

Onset: gradual, but may worsen to a medical emergency

Symptoms: extreme thirst   frequent urination
dry skin   hunger
blurry vision   drowsiness
slow healing wounds

Treatment:

- Take blood sugar reading.

- May drink water.

- Call prescriber.

- Call prescriber if blood glucose levels are higher than normal or per recommendation of DMMP.

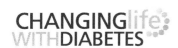
Hyperglycemia (High Blood Glucose)

Causes: Too much food, too little insulin or diabetes pills, illness, or stress.

Onset: Often starts slowly.

Some Symptoms:

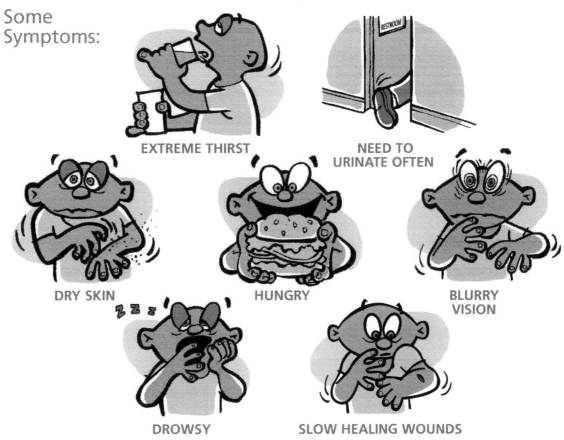

EXTREME THIRST

NEED TO URINATE OFTEN

DRY SKIN

HUNGRY

BLURRY VISION

DROWSY

SLOW HEALING WOUNDS

HIGH BLOOD GLUCOSE MAY LEAD TO A MEDICAL EMERGENCY IF NOT TREATED.

What Can You Do?

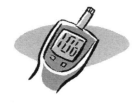

CHECK BLOOD GLUCOSE

If your blood glucose levels are higher than your goal for three days and you don't know why,

CALL YOUR HEALTHCARE PROVIDER

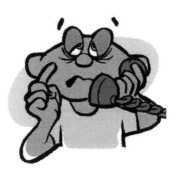

For more information, call the Novo Nordisk Tip Line at 1-800-260-3730 or visit us online at ChangingDiabetes-us.com.

© Novo Nordisk Inc.   126379R   ChangingDiabetes-us.com   6/2006   Printed in U.S.A.

novo nordisk®

The illustration below is an example of a daily routine for a client with diabetes. The goal is to maintain a blood sugar level in the proper range, which determined by the doctor's orders or DMMP (Diabetes Medication Management Plan). In the treatment of diabetes, medicine does not make it go away. The goal of medication is to control diabetes. Under the best of circumstances, adolescents must adjust to the many physical changes they undergo. Their busy lifestyle, late nights, various eating habits, up-and-down stress, and school schedules can impact blood sugar levels; therefore, staff should plan ahead and be as prepared as possible for the unexpected. Staff should also remember they are a part of a team of treatment persons with physicians and nurses available for support, questions, and guidance. Staff should make the most of those supports, refer to the American Diabetes Association, and ask questions.

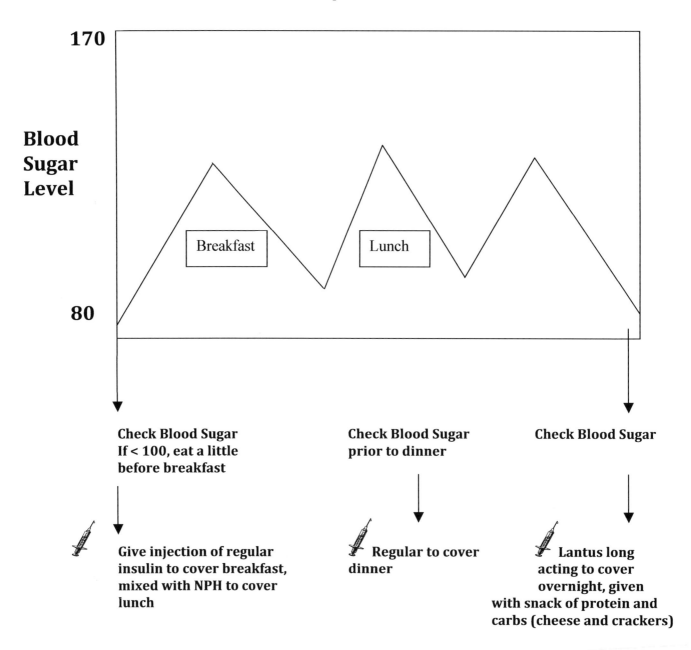

Section 28 – Facilitating a Client's Awareness of Medication Purposes and Effects

Using the information learned in this training, participants will be able to:
- effectively role play how they would explain the purpose of medication to a client;
- accurately review the prescription details to a client;
- accurately describe the three possible effects to a client: desired effects, unwanted (side) effects, and no apparent desired effect.

1. Staff should always use a supportive and patient tone when discussing medications with the client. Age appropriate language should be used that the client can understand. Staff's tone should convey the message that monitoring for medication effects will be a collaborative effort between the client and staff.

2. Staff should explain to a client that there are several reasons for prescribing medications. This overview can help the client put his or her prescription into perspective.

   a. Prevent illness such as a vaccine for various diseases or infections.
   b. Eliminate illness such as an antibiotic for infection.
   c. Control a disease such as insulin for diabetes.
   d. Reduce symptoms related to an illness such as a cold medication.
   e. Alter behavior or mood such as antidepressant, mood stabilizer, or ADHD medication.

3. Staff should then explain that the medication is intended for one of the above purposes. For example, if it is a psychotropic medication, staff would explain that the medication is intended to help improve their mood and daily functioning, or staff could explain that an antibiotic is likely to help get rid of an infection that could cause more serious problems. Staff should explain how symptoms or problems could improve with the use of the medication and possibly get worse without it.

4. Staff should then review details of the prescription with the client. A visual aid such as the prescription, the medication package, or information insert from the pharmacy could be helpful in talking with the client. A credible and established website could also facilitate reviewing medication information together.

5. Reassure the client that watching for improvement, problems, or no effect will be a collective effort with staff and the client working together.

6. Educate the client about several of the most common unwanted side effects and encourage them to self-monitor and to keep staff informed.

Section 29 – Effective Communication Among Staff

Participants will be able to:
- explain why effective communication patterns are important to good client care;
- name and explain at least 4 aspects of effective communication among staff.

Safe and competent client care requires good communication among staff. Staff must have a pattern of communication that meets particular guidelines as described below.

1. **Timely communication.** For client related information to be most useful, it needs to be current. Current documentation, for example, is essential to avoiding errors such as a staff person administering an extra dose of medication because his or her co-worker took too long to record an earlier medication administration. Progress notes, for example, that are entered late deprive staff of potentially critical information that may be needed in the upcoming hours or days. Late communications about clients make it extremely difficult to avoid preventable behavioral or medical crises. Urgent or emergency client situations are rarely predictable. Staff must develop the habit of communicating client information without delays or procrastination because it is virtually impossible to know when that information will be needed by others to provide good client care. Staff should never be in a position of saying, "I didn't know," or "I wish had known earlier."

2. **Accessible communications.** As a guideline, all staff having client care duties should have access to whatever channels of communication are used in the program to provide client information.

3. **Two-way communications.** As a guideline, effective means of communication allow staff to both receive and send, or add to the communications about clients. These two-way channels of communication help to refine the accurate pool of up-to-date client information.

4. **Communication channels that highlight client precautions.** As with any other group of people, clients routinely develop problems that deserve extra attention on a temporary basis. That category of client information needs to be highlighted in such a way that appropriate and safe precautions can be carried out by staff. For example, if a client sustains an ankle injury while playing basketball and needs to avoid activities that can worsen the injury, a communications procedure should be in place so staff can alert each other to keep the client away from sports related activities until further notice.

5. **Stored communications.** As a guideline, effective communication procedures should have the capacity to store information about clients. Sometimes the sequence of communications about clients needs to be reviewed in hindsight to diagnose and fix communication breakdowns that occur among staff or within a facility. From time to time, staff persons have the need to remind themselves of individualized client information that was announced days or weeks earlier. Good communication channels should allow for looking up archived information. Storing communications about clients is also necessary to meet various regulations.

6. **Avoid individualized communication patterns.** Over time, staff persons can develop individualized ways of communicating with each other outside the public channels of communication established by the program or facility. Although individualized channels of communication about clients might work well in the short-term for a small number of close-knit staff, it also becomes a "closed system" of communication where only that small group of staff has access to the information and how it gets exchanged. Other staff or new staff, who need the client information, would not have access. In addition, the more staff communicate with each other in a closed or idiosyncratic system, the more they tend to neglect exchanging information in the appropriate public channels of communication, which could result in poor client care.

 The role of program administrators is to establish the facility's regulations governing communication practices and to provide the resources for carrying out those practices (such as electronic communication hardware/software or paper "shift reports," for example). The role of staff is to consistently follow facility communication guidelines and to develop the effective communication behaviors described above.

Appendix 1 - Glossary of Terms

Acute Illness: a short-term and often intense illness that has a sudden onset.

Adverse Effects: a serious, unexpected and undesired reaction to medication that requires immediate intervention.

Allergic Reaction: a potentially harmful immune response to a foreign substance which could include medication. These reactions occur when the immune system overreacts to a substance called an allergen. These reactions do not always occur the first time the trigger or allergen is introduced and may worsen with each exposure to the substance.

Anaphylaxis: a severe and potentially life threatening sudden allergic reaction characterized by hives, swelling, shortness of breath, and requiring immediate treatment.

Asthma: a chronic condition characterized by severe difficulty breathing caused by a spasm of the bronchial tubes or by swelling of mucous membranes caused by a response to a trigger and/or allergen.

Auto-Injector: a device for delivering an injection by an automatic system. EpiPen® is an example of an auto-injector device for delivering epinephrine when a client has a severe allergic reaction.

Brand Name: a name given to the medicine by the pharmaceutical company that created it.

Cannula - small, stiff but flexible tubing designed to remove or administer fluids. For insulin pumps for diabetic clients, it helps deliver small continuous amounts of insulin just under the skin.

Chemical Restraint: the use of strong sedating medication to calm a client who is extremely agitated. For the purpose of working with the intended clients described in this MATY curriculum, chemical restraints are <u>never</u> permitted.

Chronic Illness: a long-term illness or disease.

Client: any individual who is provided services through your program.

Controlled Medication: a medication with a high potential for abuse, addiction and/or serious adverse effects (such as a narcotic or pain medication) that must be regulated through prescriptions and extra storage precautions.

Day School: abbreviation for "school for students with disabilities." Disabilities are generally defined as social, emotional or behavioral problems that interfere with a child's learning and functioning.

Diabetes: a metabolic disorder that leads to persistently high sugar levels in the blood.

DMMP: Diabetic Medication Management Plan – a diabetic action plan ordered by the client's insulin-prescribing health care provider.

Extrapyramidal Symptoms: involuntary motor movements (such as tremors, twitching, restlessness, or rigidity) that are mild or serious side effects of certain medications particularly antipsychotic medications.

Generic Name: the chemical name of a medication rather than the advertised brand name under which it is sold.

Glucagon: A hormone produced in the pancreas that raises the level of glucose in the blood. A glucagon injection may be given to a diabetic child in an emergency to raise exteremely low blood glucose levels.

Hyperglycemia: abnormally high blood sugar level that needs to be treated with medication/insulin, nutrition changes, and/or lifestyle changes

Insulin: a hormone secreted by the pancreas to carry blood sugar to cells. It occurs naturally, but for diabetic clients can be provided externally to help keep blood sugar within a healthy range.

Legal Guardian: the adult-aged person with legal custody of a child or adolescent client. The legal guardian is the person with the authority to accept or decline treatment for the client, and has the authority to make other decisions, such as whether the client can attend or participate in activities. The legal guardian may be a biological parent, adoptive parent, an extended family member, or a social services agency (such as a social worker employed by a county's or city's Department of Social Services), for example.

Nebulizer: a device used to administer asthma medication. It has an electronically powered compressor that forces air through the device to produce a fine medication mist that is inhaled through a mask or mouthpiece.

Nocturnal Enuresis: commonly referred to as bedwetting or nighttime urinary incontinence, nocturnal enuresis is involuntary urination while asleep by a person who is at or beyond the age in which his or her bladder would normally control such an occurrence.

OTC Medication: over-the counter medication, medication that does not usually need a prescription.

Other Medication: all prescription medications that are not controlled medications. They can be dispensed without a prescription, but clients served under the protocols of the MATY program do require a prescription. The potential for mild to serious side effects is still present in non-controlled medications.

Parent Figure: the adult-aged person who participates in the client's life as a parent. The parent figure may be a biological parent, grandparent, aunt or uncle, foster parent, adoptive parent, respite care parent or an advocate figure associated with an agency such as the Department of Social Services or the juvenile court system. The parent figure may, or may not be the legal guardian. If the parent figure is not the legal guardian, their active involvement may warrant notifying them of client health care needs and changes. If the parent figure is not legal guardian, the legal guardian's consent for staff to communicate with the parent figure about the client must be obtained. Some agencies may also use the term "**authorized representative**" – refer to your lead regulatory agency for specific guidance.

Prescriber: a licensed health care provider with advanced education who is legally authorized to prescribe medications according to state regulations and codes. The most common examples of prescribers are physicians, nurse practitioners, dentists, and psychiatrists.

PRN: "as needed" medication. Medication given to treat specific symptoms at nonspecific and/or intermittent times, often to relieve or control symptoms that may recur from a known condition. Ibuprofen for relief of intermittent pain is an example.

Protective gloves: disposable, single-use, waterproof, and latex-free or vinyl gloves.

Psychotropic Medications: medications that are used to treat psychological problems related to depression, anxiety, extreme mood swings, psychosis, hyperactivity and poor concentration.

Rights of Clients: all clients in have human rights that impact how services are provided, such as the right to refuse medication and to have their medical needs addressed in a timely manner. See page 5 for further details.

Tardive Dyskinesia: involuntary movements cased by medication side effects. A type of extrapyramidal symptoms that specifically affect the areas of the mouth, lips or tongue.

Titrate: a term used to either increase and/or decrease a medication to alleviate any potential side effects and/or to reach a therapeutic level of a medication.

 The hand symbol is used in the MATY curriculum to emphasize the extra importance of some training information and is often related to critical safety information.

 The building symbol is used in the MATY curriculum to highlight information that is closely linked to the regulations, procedures, and administrative practices of individual programs. Individual facilities can and do vary in terms of specific procedures for administering medication and meeting the health care needs of children and adolescents. Therefore it is critical MATY participants know how to apply their MATY training in their particular program.

Appendix 2 – Information and Reference Sources

<u>Medication Reference Books (Use Most Current Editions)</u>

1. "The Pill Book" by Harold M. Silverman (2012), 15th edition

2. Mosby's 2015 Nursing Drug Reference" by Linda Skidmore (2015)

3. 2015 PDR Nurse's Drug Handbook" by Physician's Desk Reference and Ivy M. Alexander

<u>Internet Reference and Resource Sites</u>

1. http://www.webmd.com/drugs/

2. http://www.rxlist.com/

3. http://www.drugs.com

4. Virginia Department of Health at http://www.vdh.virginia.gov/

5. Virginia Department of Social Services at http://www.dss.virginia.gov/

6. Centers for Disease Control and Prevention at http://www.cdc.gov/

7. Virginia Department of Education at http://www.doe.virginia.gov/

8. Virginia Board of Nursing at http://www.dhp.virginia.gov/nursing/

9. The Joint Commission at http://www.jointcommission.org/

10. The Institute for Safe Medication Practices at http://www.ismp.org/

11. American Diabetes Association at www.diabetes.org

12. American Academy of Allergy, Asthma, and Immunology www.aaaai.org

13. Virginia Board of Pharmacy at http://www.dhp.virginia.gov/Pharmacy/

14. Food and Drug Administration at http://www.fda.gov/

15. Printable medical forms at http://www.freeprintablemedicalforms.com/

Appendix 3 - Orientation Checklist for Primary Work Setting

 If training is conducted at a site other than participant's place of employment, it is recommended that they complete an orientation process at that site to translate what they have learned to their own work setting and ensure full knowledge of all program policies and procedures.

Within their primary work setting, MATY staff will be capable of answering the following questions.

1. Where are the facility's regulations and policies and procedures located, and how are they accessed?
2. What pharmacy provides services for the facility? And where is the pharmacy contact information located?
3. Who is the staff person's immediate supervisor? What is the administrative hierarchy in the program?
4. Where is contact information located for the clients' physicians, dentists and prescribers if necessary?
5. Where is contact information located for the clients' parent figures and/or legal guardians?
6. Who is the facility's primary licensing agency?
7. Where are the medication administration areas located?
8. Where are medication administration supplies located?
9. Where are the Medication Administration Records (MARs) located?
10. Where are individual client records stored, and how can those records be accessed?
11. How are client progress notes entered?
12. Where are First Aid supplies located?
13. How can past client progress notes and records be accessed and read?
14. What are the channels of communication among staff at the facility? Email versus verbal shift reports, for example?

Appendix 4 – Guidance on Annual Refresher Requirement

Although MATY certification does not expire or require retraining or recertification, the completion of an **annual refresher** is required to keep the certification in good standing. While neither the MATY curriculum, nor VAISEF offer strict requirements as to the content of these annual refreshers, it is suggested that they focus on those areas of a facility's medication administration program that have been identified throughout the year as needing improvement. While all staff and programs strive to ensure the health and well being of their clients, facilities engaging in this performance and quality improvement (PQI) process will inevitably be able to identify areas of improvement in their medication administration program.

A facility's on-going medication administration PQI process should examine areas such as:
- errors in medication administration (i.e., Six Rights of Medication Administration)
- documenting medication errors
- issues associated with medication administration records (MARs)
- medication storage
- proper labeling
- transportation of medication
- proper use/management of over-the-counter (OTC) medications
- proper disposal/destruction of medications
- staff ability to recognize the effectiveness of client's medications and knowledge of medication side-effects
- staff communication with clients, including educating clients on the purpose of their prescribed medications
- managing refusals

Facilities that go through this annual PQI process will be able to better identify those areas where MATY-trained staff need refreshing. Facilities should not, however, limit their PQI process to examining only those bulleted areas above; instead, administrators and MATY-trained staff should think in terms of examining all areas of the MATY curriculum to incorporate in their quality improvement process. This is also an opportunity to discuss any clients served whose medication administration needs are not covered by MATY.

Suggestions on how to facilitate a MATY annual refresher may include:
- Structuring the facility's refresher to include those areas identified by the facility's PQI process.
- Encouraging participants to discuss specific issues they may have encountered so the others might benefit from the real-life experiences of their colleagues.
- Post-test participants to both ensure participants continue to possess the competencies needed to properly administer the facility's medication program as well as provide the organization with documentation that they have properly trained staff administering medications. Pre-testing is also an option. Suggestions for testing content include, but are not limited to:
  - test-type questions related to those specific PQI areas that were addressed
  - questions related to the Six Rights of Medication Administration
  - have participants "set-up" a MAR from a physician's written order
  - create a test-copy MAR that contains multiple errors and have participants identify these errors and correct them

Who can facilitate MATY annual refresher?
MATY annual refreshers can only be facilitated by a MATY-trained individual or by a person otherwise licensed to administer medications (RN, LPN, MD, other licensed health care professional, or individual certified to administer medication under another program). Such individual should be familiar with the facility's policies and procedures and MATY curriculum.

What is the required length of time for the annual refresher?
While the MATY program does not require a specific length of time for the annual refresher, the length of time should be adequate enough to incorporate areas of needed focus, allow facilitator to determine participants have the knowledge they need to effectively implement the facility's medication administration program, and if applicable to the organization, allow for post-testing and feedback.

For additional questions regarding the MATY annual refresher requirement, please contact the MATY program through VAISEF at maty@vaisef.org or (804) 643-2776.

Appendix 5 - Client Documentation Descriptors

The descriptors listed below are intended to be useful examples to assist staff in communicating with others about clients. This appendix is a supplement to Section 9, Documenting Medication Administration.

Affect (Observation of Facial and Emotional Expressions)

varies appropriately	appropriate to situation	laughing
happy	upbeat	excited
animated	euphoric	euthymic (neutral, normal)
relaxed	calm	alert
expressive	limited expressiveness	constricted
flat	almost expressionless	catatonic
sadbored	confused	
melancholy	distressed	stressed
anxious	nervous	uneasy
pained	confused	intense

Energy Level

age appropriate	appropriate to situation	sluggish
listless	fatigued	low
weak	active	very active as shown by…
on the go	restless	seemed constantly on the go
frequently touching things	fidgety	jumps from project to project
talkative	interrupts others	jumps from topic to topic
asks many questions	clumsy	accident prone
loud versus soften spoken	up and down cycles	hectic or disorganized energy

Mood

appropriate to situations	varied appropriately	neutral (euthymic)
within normal limits	cooperative	friendly
gloomy in appearance	sad in appearance	hopeless
dejected in appearance	crying, tearful	quiet
irritable or touchy	agitated as shown by…	upset
grumpy	frustrated	excitable
happy	joyful	moody as shown by…
explosive	volatile	humorous or joking
euphoric	expansive	over reactive
angry as shown by…	worried	ambivalent
disinterested	distant	oppositional
defiant	argumentative	sarcastic

Appetite

within normal limits	weak	poor to extremely poor
minimal	declining over time	improving compared to…
worse compared to…	large	endless
ravenous	bottomless	healthy based on…

Sleep

undisturbed	uninterrupted	restful
no delay in sleep onset	restless	slept through the night
appears to need little sleep	wants to sleep often	delayed sleep onset (how long)

does / does not talk in sleep

does / does not have or complain of nightmares

does / does not sleepwalk

awakened during the night (once, several times, often)

awoke early and could not return to sleep despite wanting to

Thinking and Memory

alert	oriented	logical
goal directed	clear headed	attentive
quick thinking	no strange comments	unusual comments such as…
able to concentrate	distractible	poor concentration as shown by…
easily distracted	absent minded	forgetful
able to remember to…	unable to remember…	jumps from topic to topic
does not edit him/herself	impulsive talker	racing thoughts as shown by …
slow to form words	does not know date	unable to state where he/she is
good / poor historian	cannot recall details	cannot recall what was just said
suspicious thinking	preoccupations with …	anxious thoughts, such as…

All of the examples and descriptors listed above have a subjective quality to a greater or lesser degree. That subjectivity is almost unavoidable when describing human feelings, expressions, and functioning. But whenever possible, it is important for staff to be precise in communicating why a description was used for a client.

For example, if a staff person asks a client, "How are you feeling?" the staff person should communicate in his or her progress note that the client's mood was depressed <u>based on self-report when asked and based on observations of mood and affect</u>.

For example, a good and precise observation note by a staff person would state the client "<u>appeared</u> distressed most of the day, <u>based on</u> his facial expressions, his frequent and anxious questions about his next home visit, and his pacing and hand-wringing."

Appendix 6 - Sample Asthma Awareness Information Sheet

Client's Name: _____ **Date of Birth:** _____
Parent(s) or Guardian(s) Name: _____
Emergency phone numbers: Mother _____ Father _____

Primary health care provider's name: _____ **Phone:** _____
Current asthma medication: _____

Known triggers for this client's asthma (circle all that apply):

colds	mold	exercise	tree pollens
dust	strong odors	grass	flowers
excitement	weather changes	animals	smoke

foods (specify): _____
other (specify): _____

Activities for which this client has needed special attention in the past (circle all that apply)

OUTDOORS	INDOORS
Field trip to see animals	Painting or renovations
Running hard	Art projects with chalk, glue
Gardening	Pet care
Outdoor on cold or windy days	Recent pesticide application
Playing in freshly cut grass	Sitting on carpets

Others (specify): _____

Typical signs and symptoms of the client's asthma episodes (circle all that apply):

Fatigue	Breathing faster	Dark circles under eyes
Flaring nostrils	Persistent coughing	Gray or blue lips or fingernails
Difficulty playing	Difficulty eating	Difficulty drinking
Difficulty talking	Face red, pale or swollen	Wheezing
Sucking in chest/neck	Mouth open (panting)	Agitation
Grunting	Restlessness	Complains of chest pain or tightness

Others (specify): _____

Remember to always bring fast-acting asthma medication with the client during off-site activities. If severe sudden asthma problem persists or worsens after fast-acting medication is administered as prescribed, seek emergency medical assistance.

Parent/Guardian Signature: _____ Date: _____

Appendix 7 - List of "Do Not Use" Abbreviations

Do Not Use	Potential Problem	Use Instead
U (unit)	Mistaken for zero, the number four or cc	Write "Unit"
IU (International Unit)	Mistaken for IV (intravenous) or the number ten	Write "International Unit"
Q.D., QD, q.d. (daily) Q.O.D., QOD, q.o.d., qod (every other day)	Mistaken for each other Period after the Q mistaken for "I" and "O" mistaken for "I"	Write "daily" Write "every other day"
Trailing zero (X.0 mg) for medication documentation. Lack of leading zero (.X mg)	Decimal point is missed	Write X mg Write 0.X mg
MS MSO$_4$ and MgSO$_4$	Can mean morphine sulfate or magnesium sulfate. Confused for one another.	Write "morphine sulfate" Write "magnesium sulfate"

Possible Future Inclusion in the "Do Not Use List"	Potential Problem	Use Instead
> (greater than) < (less than)	Misinterpreted as the number seven or the letter "L"	Write "greater than" Write "less than"
Abbreviations for medication names	Misinterpreted due to similar abbreviations for multiple medications	Write medication names in full
@	Mistaken for the number two	Write "at"
cc (for cubic centimeter)	Mistaken for U (units) when poorly written	Write "mL" or "ml" or "milliliters" ("mL" is preferred)
µg (for microgram)	Mistaken for mg (milligrams) resulting in one thousand-fold overdose	Write "mcg" or "micrograms"

Possible Future Inclusion in the "Do Not Use List"	Potential Problem	Use Instead
T.I.W. (three times a week)	Mistaken for three times a day or twice weekly resulting in an overdose	Write "3 times weekly" or "three times weekly"
A.S. (left ear) A.D. (right ear) A.U. (both ears) O.S. (left eye) O.D. (right eye) O.U. (both eyes)	Mistaken for each other	Write "left ear" Write "right ear" Write "both ears" Write "left eye" Write "right eye" Write "both eyes"

Most of the information for this appendix is from The Joint Commission website and their "Do Not Use" list as of June 2009.

Additional abbreviations were included from the Institute for Safe Medication Practices (ISMP) website as of June 2009.

Appendix 8 – Medicines Recommended for Disposal By Flushing

Listed by Medicine and Active Ingredient
List Revised: February 2015

There is a small number of medicines that may be especially harmful and, in some cases, fatal with just one dose if they are used by someone other than the person for whom the medicine was prescribed. This list from FDA tells you what expired, unwanted, or unused medicines you should flush down the sink or toilet to help prevent danger to people and pets in the home.

FDA continually evaluates medicines for safety risks and will update the list as needed. Please visit the Disposal of Unused Medicines: What You Should Know page at www.fda.gov for more information.

Medicine	Active Ingredient
Abstral, tablets (sublingual)	Fentanyl
Actiq, oral transmucosal lozenge *	Fentanyl Citrate
Avinza, capsules (extended release)	Morphine Sulfate
Buprenorphine Hydrochloride, tablets (sublingual) *	Buprenorphine Hydrochloride
Buprenorphine Hydrochloride; Naloxone Hydrochloride, tablets (sublingual) *	Buprenorphine Hydrochloride; Naloxone Hydrochloride
Butrans, transdermal patch system	Buprenorphine
Daytrana, transdermal patch system	Methylphenidate
Demerol, tablets *	Meperidine Hydrochloride
Demerol, oral solution *	Meperidine Hydrochloride
Diastat/Diastat AcuDial, rectal gel	Diazepam
Dilaudid, tablets *	Hydromorphone Hydrochloride
Dilaudid, oral liquid *	Hydromorphone Hydrochloride
Dolophine Hydrochloride, tablets *	Methadone Hydrochloride
Duragesic, patch (extended release) *	Fentanyl
Embeda, capsules (extended release)	Morphine Sulfate; Naltrexone Hydrochloride
Exalgo, tablets (extended release)	Hydromorphone Hydrochloride
Fentora, tablets (buccal)	Fentanyl Citrate
Hysingla ER, tablets (extended release)	Hydrocodone Bitartrate

Medicine	Active Ingredient
Kadian, capsules (extended release)	Morphine Sulfate
Methadone Hydrochloride, oral solution *	Methadone Hydrochloride
Methadose, tablets *	Methadone Hydrochloride
Morphine Sulfate, tablets (immediate release) *	Morphine Sulfate
Morphine Sulfate, oral solution *	Morphine Sulfate
MS Contin, tablets (extended release) *	Morphine Sulfate
Nucynta ER, tablets (extended release)	Tapentadol
Onsolis, soluble film (buccal)	Fentanyl Citrate
Opana, tablets (immediate release)	Oxymorphone Hydrochloride
Opana ER, tablets (extended release)	Oxymorphone Hydrochloride
Oxecta, tablets (immediate release)	Oxycodone Hydrochloride
Oxycodone Hydrochloride, capsules	Oxycodone Hydrochloride
Oxycodone Hydrochloride, oral solution	Oxycodone Hydrochloride
Oxycontin, tablets (extended release)	Oxycodone Hydrochloride
Percocet, tablets *	Acetaminophen; Oxycodone Hydrochloride
Percodan, tablets *	Aspirin; Oxycodone Hydrochloride
Suboxone, film (sublingual)	Buprenorphine Hydrochloride; Naloxone Hydrochloride
Xartemis XR tablets	Oxycodone Hydrochloride; Acetaminophen
Xyrem, oral solution	Sodium Oxybate
Zohydro ER capsules (extended release)	Hydrocodone Bitartrate
Zubsolv tablets (sublingual)	Buprenorphine Hydrochloride; Naloxone Hydrochloride

These medicines have generic versions available or are only available in generic formulations.

Appendix 9 – Sample Severe Allergy Action Plan

Student Name: _____

DOB: _____ Date: _____ Grade/Homeroom: _____

PHYSICIAN ORDERS/PLAN OF CARE

Health Care Provider _____ _____ _____

                                     Printed Name   Signature   Date

                                     _____   _____

                                     Provider Phone   Provider Fax

ALLERGY TO: _____

High risk for severe reaction:	YES___	NO____
History of Asthma:	YES ___	NO ____
Asthma Action Plan:	YES ____	NO ___

MEDICATION ORDERED FOR ALLERGY SYMPTOMS (please complete symptom checklist below)

1. Antihistamine: Benadryl/Diphenhydramine HCL:_____mg/Other:_____
2. Inhaler: Medication _____Dose_____/Follow Asthma Action Plan YES NO
3. Epinephrine Auto Injector (Junior) 0.15mg Epinephrine Auto Injector 0.30mg
4. Repeat Epinephrine Auto Injector: NO YES, when_____
5. Other:_____

Symptoms Give Checked Medication

	Epi pen	Antihistamine
--If insect stings, but NO SYMPTOMS	☐ Epi pen	☐ Antihistamine
--If a food allergen has been ingested, but NO	☐ Epi pen	☐ Antihistamine
--MOUTH: itching/tingling/swelling of lips, tongue, mouth	☐ Epi pen	☐ Antihistamine
--SKIN: hives, itching, swelling about the extremities	☐ Epi pen	☐ Antihistamine
--GI: nausea, abdominal cramps, vomiting and/or diarrhea	☐ Epi pen	☐ Antihistamine
--LUNGS: shortness of breath, repetitive cough, wheezing	☐ Epi pen	☐ Antihistamine
--HEART: thready pulse, low blood pressure, fainting	☐ Epi pen	☐ Antihistamine
--OTHER: _____	☐ Epi pen	☐ Antihistamine

***The severity of these symptoms can change quickly and progress rapidly to a life-threatening situation**

1. Give medications as ordered above. Note time medications given.
2. Monitor student and instruct someone to CALL 911 (if Epinephrine is given, or as needed).
3. Notify parent/guardian and school administrator.
4. Additional instructions/orders:

_____

_____   _____   _____

Parent/Guardian Signature   **Parent Printed Name**   **Date**

Appendix 10 - Sample Daily Record of Insulin Administrations

Daily Record of Insulin Administrations

Date	Time	Amount of Insulin	Blood Glucose Level	Injection Site

Notes: _____

_____

_____

_____

_____

_____

_____

Appendix 11 - Sample Daily Count Sheet for Controlled Medications

Client's Controlled Medication Record

Client Name	Facility/Program Name	Physician / Prescriber			
Medication Name	Dosage	Instructions for Administration			

Name of Staff Administering	Date	Time	Amount On Hand	Amount Received	Amount Given	Amount Remaining

Appendix 12 – Samples of Medication Administration Records

PRN MEDICATION ADMINISTRATION RECORD

Student Name: _____   **Allergies:** _____

School Year: 2008 - 2009   **DOB:** _____

Medication (dose, route, measure)											
Acetaminophen (Tylenol: Reg Strength) 650 mg, p.o., 2 tabs	Date										
	Time										
	Initials										
	Date										
	Time										
	Initials										
	Date										
	Time										
	Initials										
	Date										
	Time										
	Initials										

STAFF AUTHORIZATION

Initials	Staff Signature	Initials	Staff Signature

MEDICATION ADMINISTRATION RECORD

Student Name: _____   DOB: _____

Allergies: _____   School Year: _____

Medication *(dose, time, frequency, route)*													
	Date/time												
	Code												
	Initials per Distribution												
	Reported Side Effects												
	Date/time												
	Code												
	Initials per Distribution												
	Reported Side Effects												
	Date/time												
	Code												
	Initials per Distribution												
	Reported Side Effects												
	Date/time												
	Code												
	Initials per Distribution												
	Reported Side Effects												

CODES

P = Planned   **A** = Absent   **X** = Not applicable   **L** = Arrived after time   **D** = Dismissed before time   **S** = Suspended   **R** = Refused
NS = No School/Holiday   **NMA** = No Medication Available   **MLOA** = Medical Leave of Absence   **MDC** = Medication Discontinued per Physician
SDC = Student Discharged/ Withdrawn   **ME** = Medication Error   **F** = Off Grounds Administration

ADVERSE SIDE EFFECTS OR REPORTED COMPLAINT

Ag=Agitation   **An**=Anxiety   **Di**=Dizziness   **Dr**=Drowsiness   **DM**=Dry Mouth   **Ha**=Hallucination   **He**=Headache   **In**=Indigestion
IA=Increased Appetite   **IH**=Irregular Heartbeat   **LA**=Lack of Appetite   **Ra**=Rash   **Re**=Restlessness   **Vo**=Vomiting   **O**=Other

STAFF AUTHORIZATION			
Initials	*Staff Signature*	*Initials*	*Staff Signature*

June 2009

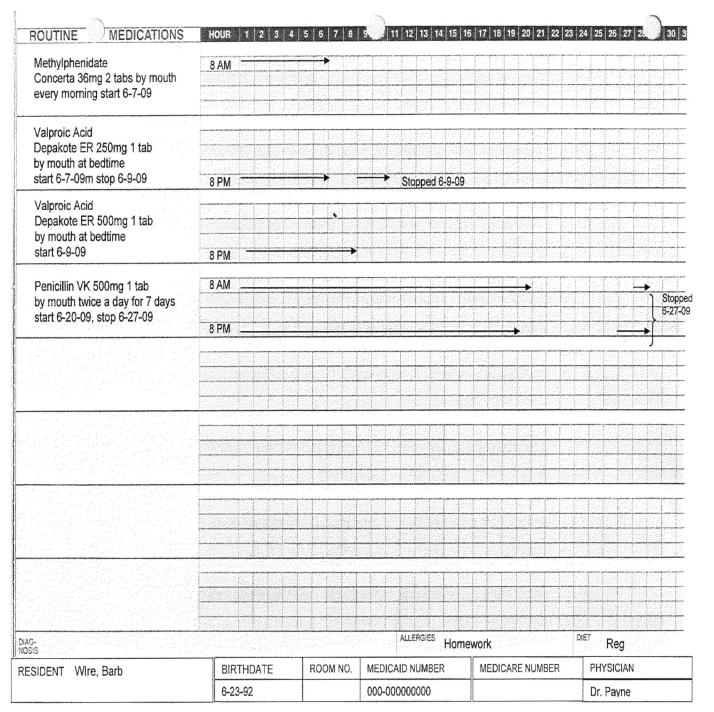

ROUTINE MEDICATIONS	HOUR	1	2	3	4	5	6	7	8	9	11	12	13	14	15	16	17	18	19	20	21	22	23	24	25	26	27	28	30	3
Methylphenidate Concerta 36mg 2 tabs by mouth every morning start 6-7-09	8 AM							→																						
Valproic Acid Depakote ER 250mg 1 tab by mouth at bedtime start 6-7-09m stop 6-9-09	8 PM					→			→	Stopped 6-9-09																				
Valproic Acid Depakote ER 500mg 1 tab by mouth at bedtime start 6-9-09	8 PM							→																						
Penicillin VK 500mg 1 tab by mouth twice a day for 7 days start 6-20-09, stop 6-27-09	8 AM																			→					→		Stopped 6-27-09		
	8 PM																			→					→				

DIAG-NOSIS

ALLERGIES Homework   DIET Reg

RESIDENT Wlre, Barb	BIRTHDATE	ROOM NO.	MEDICAID NUMBER	MEDICARE NUMBER	PHYSICIAN
	6-23-92		000-000000000		Dr. Payne

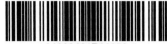

Made in the USA
Middletown, DE
01 October 2018